THE
YOGA
DIRECTORY

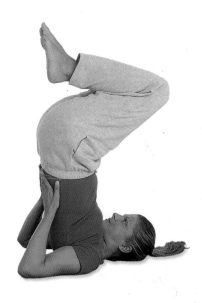

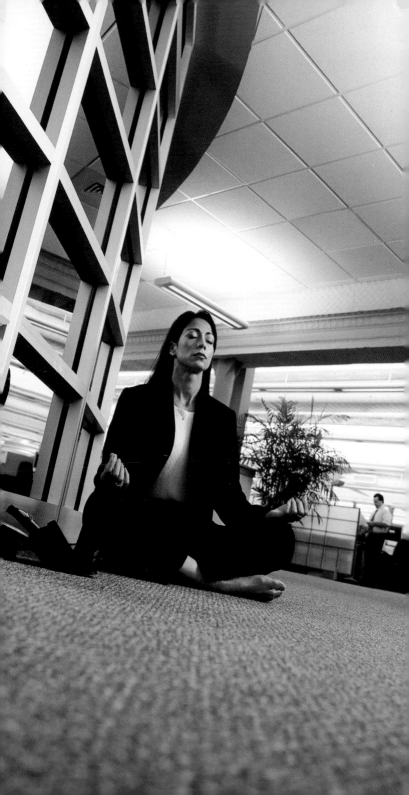

Linda Doeser

THE
YOGA
DIRECTORY

METRO BOOKS
NEW YORK

Note from the publisher
This book should be considered as a reference source only and it
is not intended to replace instruction or advice from a qualified
practitioner or other healthcare professional. The author and
publisher disclaim any liability, loss, injury, or damage incurred
as a consequence, directly or indirectly, of the use and
application of the contents.

This book was conceived, designed, and produced by
Ivy Press
The Old Candlemakers, West Street,
Lewes, East Sussex, BN7 2NZ, UK

CREATIVE DIRECTOR Peter Bridgewater
PUBLISHER Sophie Collins
EDITORIAL DIRECTOR Steve Luck
DESIGN MANAGER Tony Seddon
DESIGNER Alistair Plumb
SENIOR PROJECT EDITOR Rebecca Saraceno
STUDIO PHOTOGRAPHY Calvey Taylor-Haw
YOGA CONSULTANT Joanne Avison

Metro Books
122 Fifth Avenue
New York, NY 10011

ISBN-13: 978-1-4351-0882-0
ISBN-10: 1-4351-0882-5

Printed in China

1 3 5 7 9 10 8 6 4 2

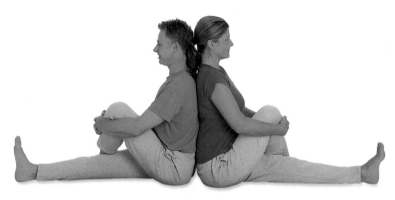

Contents

Introduction

While it is no surprise that India's national cricket team practices yoga, the number of Westerners who have taken it up is astonishing. It is arguably the fastest-growing fitness activity in the West. Undoubtedly, this is in part due to fashion—just like the explosion of interest in aerobics some decades earlier, high-profile stars and celebrities have boosted its popularity. But the secret of yoga's success stems from something far deeper and longer-lasting.

Yoga is not simply another form of exercise, although many people do take it up because they want to acquire stronger, more supple, and shapelier bodies. Rather, it is a system of physical and spiritual techniques for achieving balance and harmony within yourself and with others and your environment. While there is no need to follow the more mystical pathways, you will find that yoga differs from other forms of exercise simply because the postures link the physical with the spiritual.

Worth noting too, though, is that yoga is very gentle; you do not have to drive yourself to raise increasingly heavy weights or double the number of push-ups. Quite the opposite—

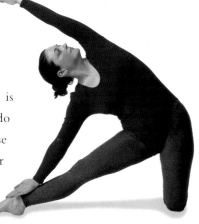

in fact, you could say, "If you feel pain, there's no gain." You learn at the pace that suits you. This is not only a reassuring approach for beginners, it is also invaluable for competitive high-achievers who need relief from constant pressure.

Some kinds of training result in highly developed muscles, which, if not constantly worked on, will turn to fat. Many sports exercise only one or two parts of the body, and this can cause irregular muscle development, strains, and injuries. Retired professional golfers, for example, often suffer from impaired shoulder movement, while urban joggers may do irreparable damage to the leg and foot joints. Yoga poses—based on a system of stretches, balances, twists, and bends—exercise the entire body. What's more, every forward movement is balanced by a backward one, and every twist to the left is countered by one to the right, so no single set of muscles is overstretched. In addition, yoga works on more than just muscles—the spine becomes more elastic, the joints loosen, the lungs expand, the circulation is stimulated, and stamina increases.

Finally, yoga is controlled and disciplined. To practice the poses, you need to focus your mind, and this has a deeply calming effect. Racing thoughts are stilled, anxiety is reduced, and stress eased.

About This Book

Like yoga itself, you can dip into this directory for aspects that are specific to your needs. The first chapter introduces some of the underlying philosophy, and places yoga in both its historical and contemporary contexts. Outlining some of the different yoga paths, it summarizes the wide range of techniques that may be followed—wholly, in part, or not at all—to achieve a sense of well-being and spiritual balance. It offers guidelines on what benefits you can derive and helpful hints for beginners on getting started. Perhaps the only piece of "required reading" is the list of contraindications (*see pages 36–37*). This list explains which poses to avoid if you are suffering from certain medical conditions. The heart of the book lies in the next two chapters, which describe both traditional classic and popular Western poses. This section

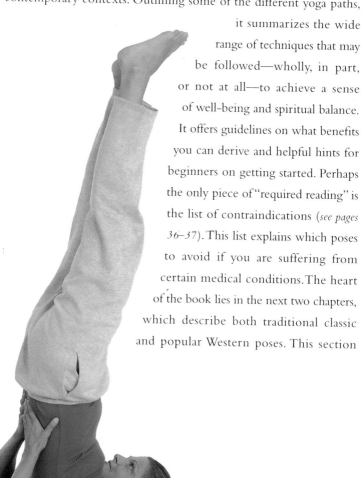

starts as you should—with warming-up exercises—and then describes individual poses in detail, offering clear step-by-step pictures and instructions. Advice is given on the benefits to be derived from each pose, and many pages include tips to help beginners when they are first learning. Each pose is graded with blue for beginners, green for intermediate, and red for advanced—but this is not absolute, because only you can estimate the scope, suppleness, and strength of your body. These two chapters do not comprise a course, and you can pick and choose which poses you want to try.

The fourth chapter presents some guidelines for regular practice and suggests

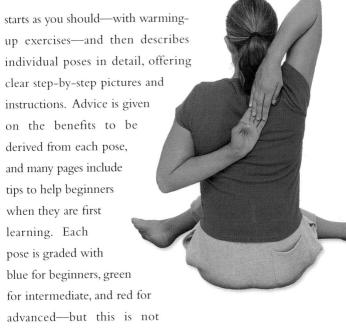

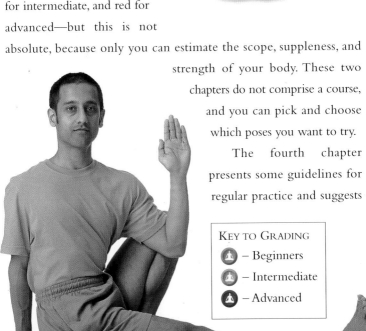

KEY TO GRADING
 – Beginners
 – Intermediate
 – Advanced

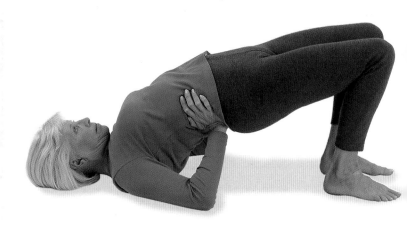

series of programs based on the poses described earlier. While all the programs have been planned to include a full range of stretches, bends, spinal twists, limb limbering, and inverted positions, they are very flexible and you can adapt them to suit your needs. The programs become successively more challenging, but there is no need to feel that you have to work through all of them. Throughout the book, the emphasis is on learning and working at your own pace.

The final chapter is full of ideas about using yoga and adapting its techniques to fit your lifestyle and to overcome some of the strains and stresses of everyday life, from sitting in a traffic jam to preventing repetitive strain injury at the computer keyboard.

How you use *The Yoga Directory* is up to you. I hope that it proves a useful map as you explore this unique path to physical and mental well-being, and hope too that you enjoy the journey. In the words of the French author Felix Guyot, when writing on yoga and health, "Keep well, remain young a long time, and live to a good old age."

LINDA DOESER

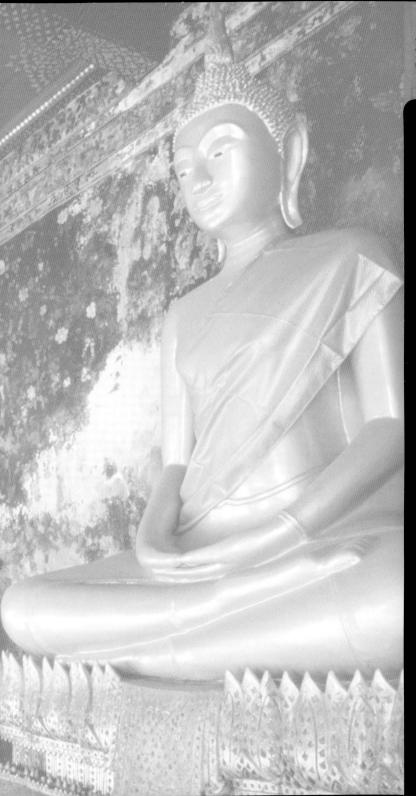

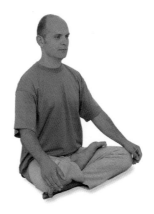

Why Yoga?

"Man's quest for perfection consists in organizing the things of body, mind, and soul into a whole."

The word *yoga* comes from Sanskrit, one of the world's oldest languages, and means union. It is a system of integrating and balancing body, mind, emotion, and spirit. Widely practiced in the East for thousands of years, it aroused little interest in the West until the twentieth century. Today some practice it as a spiritual pathway, and others as a form of gentle exercise, and it is a popular way of relieving that great Western disease, stress. Whatever the reason, yoga brings its myriad benefits to all.

What Is Yoga?

When Westerners think of yoga, their minds usually turn first to the postures or poses known as *asanas*. In fact, these form only one aspect of yoga, although they are a significant pathway toward the ultimate goal of physical, mental, and spiritual union. They are a means of disciplining the body and were developed to balance the body's energies to free the mind to meditate. In the philosophy of yoga, they are not an end in themselves, just one of several routes toward spiritual enlightenment. This kind of physical yoga, known as *Hatha*, is one of five main paths. The others are known as *Karma*, *Jnana* (sometimes spelled *Gyana*), *Bhakti* (sometimes spelled *Bakti*), and *Raja*.

Karma is described as the yoga of action, but "action" in this context is spiritual rather than physical. Practitioners seek to eliminate their own ego and selflessly serve humanity. In rather oversimplified terms, this path to enlightenment lies in good deeds without expectation of reward.

Jnana is the yoga of philosophy. Spiritual wisdom is sought through rigorous intellectual techniques and meditation. The mind is used to penetrate the veils of illusion, which cloud the real world and the true self.

Practitioners of the yoga of devotion, Bhakti, dedicate themselves to a life of prayer and spiritual growth. This pathway transmutes human emotions through prayers, praise, mantras (incantations), and rites into divine love.

Raja is the yoga of science—in its Eastern rather than Western sense. Meditation is used as a means of purifying and controlling the mind, linking directly with both inner and outer truths and, ultimately, achieving union with the universe.

There are other forms of yoga, such as Yantra and Tantric, and different kinds overlap. Hatha, for example, is a form of Raja yoga, although some people prefer to concentrate on the physicality of the asanas, rather than the spiritual aspects of meditation. Equally, many people develop their own system of yoga, incorporating aspects of several pathways. In fact, it could be said that any of the forms of yoga will almost inevitably incorporate elements from them all.

Hatha is the best-known form of yoga in the West.

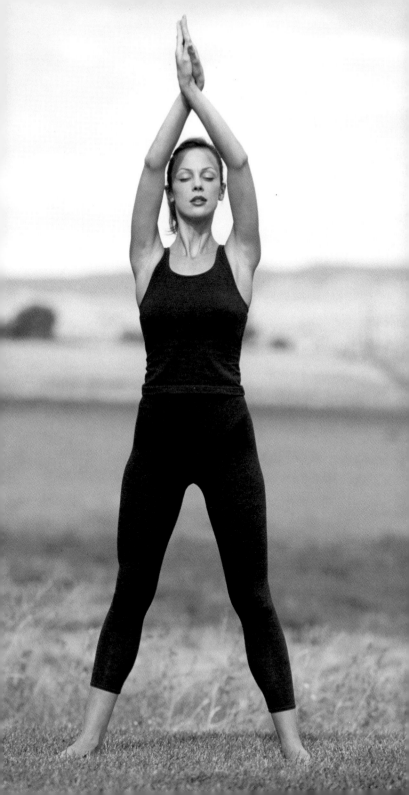

What's in It for You?

Most Westerners approach yoga for one of two motives—spiritual or physical—which, in a characteristically Western fashion, are often seen as opposing. Even the briefest study of the subject quickly reveals that the opposite is true: the beginner, concentrating on only one aspect, will soon derive benefits that connect to other pathways.

That said, Hatha yoga is the most popular type in the West and is the focus of this book. At its most basic, practicing the poses on a regular basis will tone the body, build stamina, and invigorate the system. These are goals worth achieving and can benefit most people. However, in the process of regular practice, you will probably discover a number of beneficial side effects, and any one of these can also be a primary goal.

Stress is an endemic problem in modern life and people resort to many techniques for overcoming it—from flopping down in front of the television with a stiff drink to a ferocious workout in the gym. However, provided you don't let the discipline of yoga—and it is a discipline—become yet another trigger for stress in your life, it can offer both relaxation and a sense of tranquillity that counterbalance daily wear and tear on a long-term basis. Learning the breathing techniques of yoga, called *pranayama* (*see pages 42–45*) is an invaluable way to deal with stressful situations, from overwork to road rage.

Yoga is not just for the young and fit. As a gentle form of exercise, it can delay many of the signs of aging and help you feel, as well as look, better. It stimulates the system, helping to maintain hormone levels and metabolic rate, and practicing pranayama has a tonic effect.

The holistic nature of yoga makes it a safe option for alleviating some common ailments, although there are a few provisos (*see pages 36–37*). It can help with a wide range of problems, such as PMS, arthritis, insomnia, backache, and, above all, any symptoms arising from poor posture. For many sufferers, it is a helpful way of tackling such conditions as insomnia and fatigue.

Tantric yoga (*see page 18*) is based on the philosophy of transforming sexual energy into spiritual energy. It is not simply a way of developing a more physically satisfying sexual relationship; it also raises the consciousness of both partners and creates harmony in the relationship.

Many people who first took up Hatha yoga solely for its physical benefits have been inspired to explore some other yoga pathways, particularly the meditation of Raja yoga. Others, especially those who are always on the go, have looked at Karma yoga and discovered new ways of approaching their work and day-to-day lives. In short, what's in it for you is that you can gain whatever benefits you want—and you have nothing to lose.

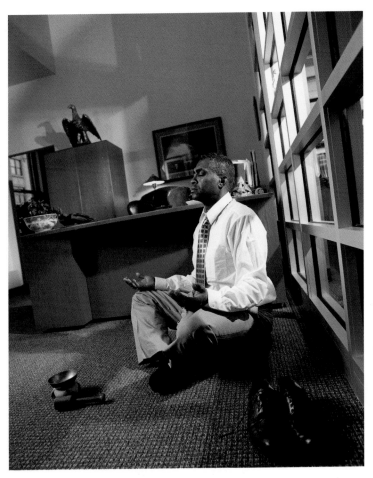

Yoga is the perfect antidote to the stress of modern life.

Where It All Began

The oldest surviving documentary evidence of what is now thought of as yoga is from the Indian subcontinent and dates from the first millennium BCE, although archeologists in India have found older artifacts depicting yoga poses. However, scholars think that these may represent a relatively advanced stage of development in a philosophy that had its origins in Southwest Asia more than 3,000 years ago.

Raja Yoga

At some time before 1000 BCE, mystics began a search for *Brahman* and *Atman* and for a way of uniting the two. Brahman is a concept of oneness; for some people, this means a supreme being or, more abstractly, the divine, while others interpret it as the cosmos. Atman is the self in a state of pure consciousness, having let go of the ego. Using meditation, often in a cross-legged or lotus position, to seek this spiritual unity is the earliest known form of yoga—Raja—and is thought to have

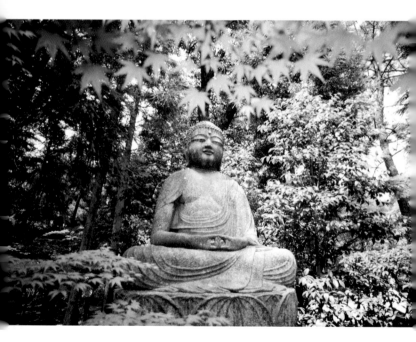

been brought to India from Persia. The sage Gautama Buddha (ca. 563–483 BCE) is frequently depicted meditating, using the techniques of Raja yoga.

The sage Patanjali, who is often called the Father of Yoga, was not its inventor, but the first to present Raja yoga systematically in the *Yoga Sutras*, written during the third and second centuries BCE. He defined yoga as "the control of the thought waves of the mind." *Sutra* means thread and describes an explanatory technique of a series of highly condensed statements, tightly packed with significance, that are joined by a thread to outline an entire philosophy. As printing did not exist, these had to be memorized, so anything that the student could be expected to know already, or infer, was left out to condense the statements as much as possible. The logic of the "thread" is often very obscure, which means that the *Yoga Sutras* are extremely difficult, for Westerners in particular, to follow. Fortunately, most translations supply detailed notes and commentaries.

Jnana Yoga

About 900 BCE, philosophers wrote the *Upanishads*, texts intended both to educate and quieten the mind. These formulate the philosophical path, or Jnana yoga, which uses the intellect and the power of reason to penetrate the veils of illusion, *Maya*, to find what is called "the space within the heart," or pure consciousness and universal oneness. It is an intellectually rigorous discipline and is generally considered the most difficult of the yoga pathways.

Karma Yoga

The active yoga path, Karma, first appeared in about 300 BCE in the poem the *Bhagavad Gita* (Song of the Lord), written by the sage Vyasa. It is based on the universal law of karma—that good actions have good results and evil actions have evil results—but places heavy and constant emphasis on the detachment of the self. While it advocates periods of contemplation and meditation, it also incorporates these processes of mental cleansing in the practice of action.

Many ancient statues of Buddha depict him in the Lotus position, the classic pose for meditation.

Tantric Yoga

In the fourth century CE, the Buddhist sage Asanga developed his philosophy of harnessing the energy of the senses and imagination to achieve a higher consciousness and, eventually, enlightenment. Some people have since misinterpreted Tantrism, whether the Buddhist or Hindu version, as a license for sexual indulgence. However, works on the philosophy—the *Tantras*—are mainly concerned with rituals, mantras, and the construction of *mandalas* (the circular symbol of unity and wholeness). Anyone looking for a cheap thrill will be disappointed by the six percent or so of material that is specifically sexual.

Bhakti Yoga

Developing to some extent from the Raja and Karma paths, Bhakti or devotional yoga was formulated by the sage Ramanuja in about CE 1000–1200. Indeed, several discourses, particularly the twelfth, of the *Bhagavad Gita* (*see page 17*) are concerned with devotional yoga and are highly regarded by practitioners of Bhakti. Prayer, songs of praise, mantras, and meditation are used as ways of uniting Brahman and Atman and achieving enlightenment. As with all yoga paths, the detachment of the self is central, so prayers are informed by pure love, rather than petitions, and mantras must have intent, rather than be mere empty repetition. Without this detachment of self, pure devotion can degenerate into hysteria—manifest as speaking in tongues, rolling in ecstasy, or even foaming at the mouth. The purity of Bhakti love is seen as a flame that burns away destructive emotions, such as anger and hatred. It is the least popular yoga path in the West, but the most popular in India.

Hatha Yoga

The last of the great classic yoga paths was developed in about CE 1000. *Ha* means sun and *tha* means moon. These symbolize the masculine and feminine energies that are encapsulated in everyone, and which must be in harmony and

Hatha yoga developed from the meditative techniques of Raja yoga as well as the physical poses of Tantric.

balance to achieve oneness. Hatha developed from the meditative techniques of Raja and the physical exercises of Tantric yoga. It was the first form to recognize asanas, and to incorporate a range of other techniques, from breathing to visualization, into a single discipline. The classic texts on Hatha yoga, mainly written in the fifteenth century, are condensed and hard to follow, rather like the *Yoga Sutras*, but translations usually include commentaries. Svatmarama's *Hatha Yoga Pradipika* is considered the standard work.

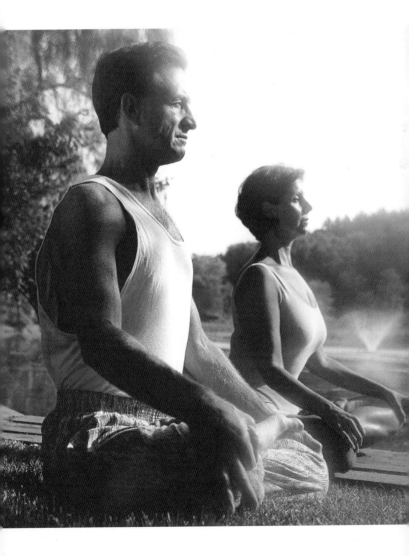

The Eight Limbs

Yoga is an integrated discipline. Even if you plan to use it only to achieve certain specific goals, you may still benefit from taking an overview, which may give you further ideas and insights. In the *Yoga Sutras*, Patanjali devised the *ashangas*, eight steps for controlling the mind. Hatha yoga emphasizes asanas and pranayama, but, strictly speaking, should also embrace the other six steps.

(1) Yamas—Abstinences

This ethical code offers five guides to abstinence: you should abstain from killing, lying, theft, sensual indulgence, and greed. However, as with all Patanjali's writings, this is more complex than it first appears. Rather than negatives—don't do this—they are positives of "not-doing."

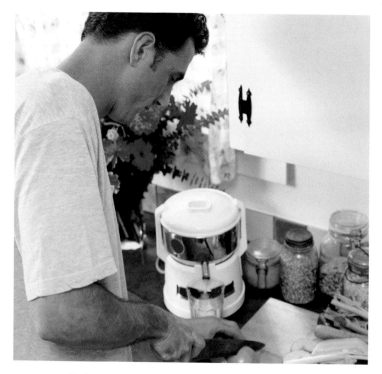

The importance of purity in yoga also relates to diet and hygiene.

If you substitute "be non-violent" for "abstain from killing," this incorporates avoiding committing any form of injury or harm, whether in word and thought, or by your actions. It also implies a positive compassion for all living creatures. Truthfulness is more than not telling lies. It also involves living with integrity and sincerity. Non-stealing, of course, means that you should not take someone else's possessions, but it also means that you should not take credit for other's work or ideas. Self-restraint can imply chastity, but this applies only to advanced students studying with a guru and not to ordinary people. Rather, it concerns avoiding excess and being moderate in all sensuous pleasures, including sexuality. Non-acquisitiveness means not defining yourself by your possessions, rather than not having any possessions at all, and suggests not being envious of other people's things or achievements. It can also include a positive generosity, not only with money, but with time and kindness.

(2) Niyamas—Observances

Observing these five qualities is a guide for personal conduct: purity, contentment, austerity, study, and resignation to Isvara (God). Again, Patanjali is condensing complex ideas into simple terms.

Purity of mind and body are much emphasized in the writings on and the practice of yoga. Should you wish to follow them, there are many guidelines on hygiene and diet (*see pages 38–41*), while assiduous practice of the asanas and pranayama help to purify the inner self. Contentment—rising above your objects of desire and cultivating tranquillity and equanimity—brings peace of mind. Austerity is sometimes translated as mortification but both terms are somewhat misleading. While fasting once a week is recommended (although it is not appropriate for everyone), this observance is more to do with strength of character and being purposeful, even in adversity, than it is with self-mortification and asceticism. Study recommends careful reading of the classic texts of yoga, but also implies self-study as a means toward achieving perfect consciousness. The final observance refers to devotion, either to a personal deity or to universal consciousness, again implying the surrender of the ego.

(3) Asanas and (4) Pranayama—
Steady Poses and Yoga Breathing

Patanjali was writing about Raja yoga, where the poses are seated ones suitable for meditation. Regulating the breath means reducing it to an appropriate level of quietness and smoothness. Both asanas and pranayama are discussed in more detail later.

(5) Pratyahara—Withdrawal of the Senses

This is the process of shutting out the stimuli that continuously bombard the senses, then shutting down the senses to turn the attention inward. It is less essential for Westernized Hatha than for Raja yoga, but proper posture and breathing, which help filter touch and smell, are essential to both.

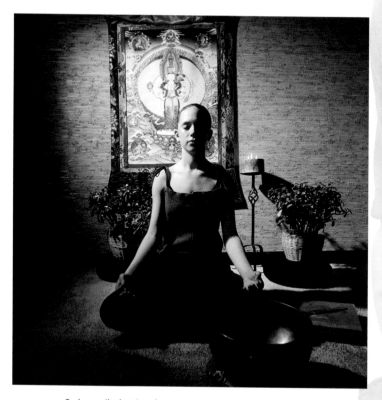

During meditation there is no past or future, only an eternal present.

(6) Dharana—Concentration

Fixing the mind on something is necessary after the shutting out of the external world. When people first start meditating, they are often surprised by the turbulence of their inner world and their whirling thoughts. One way to practice meditation is to focus your attention on a small object, such as a flower, candle flame, or yantra (symbolic design), placed a short distance away. Alternatively, shut your eyes and concentrate on a mantra or chant. 'Om' (*see page 33*) is the best-known and the most helpful for beginners. Train your mind, like a spotlight, on your chosen object. A similar beaming of attention can also be helpful when you are learning new poses, especially some of the more advanced ones.

(7) Dhyana—Meditation

This step follows naturally from Dharana, as the mind becomes conscious only of itself and the object on which it is focussed. With practice, you will be able to maintain this mental equilibrium without any further effort.

PHYSICAL AND EMOTIONAL BENEFITS

- Increases stamina
- Re-energizes the body
- Helps relaxation
- Relieves insomnia
- Reduces stress and anxiety
- Reduces blood pressure, slowing the heart rate
- Lowers breathing rate
- Increases personal space
- Clears the mind
- Reduces emotional confusion and turmoil
- Restores balance and lightens the spirit
- Assists in breaking bad habits, such as smoking
- Recharges the batteries

(8) Samadhi—Enlightenment

This is the last state in controlling "the thought waves of the mind," whereby the person meditating, the focus of attention, and the process of meditation merge and unite. It may be described as a state of super-consciousness or self-realization.

Hidden Benefits

The eight limbs, with their emphasis on controlling the mind, may seem to have no relevance for anyone using yoga simply to exercise. You may not be interested in finding your inner reality or even convinced that it exists. However, don't dismiss these steps—they have many benefits on a physical and emotional level.

The Journey from the East

India was the jewel in the crown of the British Empire and, during the nineteenth century, Western scholars and academics belatedly turned their attention toward the venerable cultural history of the subcontinent. Ancient texts, including the *Upanishads*, the *Bhagavad Gita,* and the *Yoga Sutras*, were translated and studied, and, in the process, yoga made its first tentative migrations to the West.

Eastern philosophies were so very different from Western religions and culture that few people, other than scholars, were remotely interested in trying to understand the true nature of yoga. No doubt, this attitude was exacerbated by the then popular notion of racial superiority. It was, perhaps, inevitable that Hatha yoga, with its emphasis on asanas, was the first of the classic schools to be publicized and, literally, put on display. The general public regarded it as a kind of Barnum and Bailey freak show, from which it derived a great deal of ill-natured amusement. In the 1890s a prize of £500 ($750), a sizeable sum then, was offered to anyone who could "emulate the fearful and wonderful contortions" of an adept visiting London, who was currently "giving a performance" of asanas an unbelievable 60 or more times a day.

Following this false start, the West gradually began to explore the philosophy and practice of yoga. Only a decade later, Paramahansa Yogananda, author of *Autobiography of a Yogi*, was welcomed to and honored in the United States. Travel broadens the mind, even in wartime, and by 1945 many people who would normally never have left their own shores had visited almost every corner of the globe, including India.

In the postwar world, people sought new meanings and new beginnings, some of them traveling to India in search of spiritual enlightenment and the healing powers of yoga. Indian teachers also traveled to the West. One of the most influential figures was B. K. S. Iyengar, who created his own system of yoga, marrying traditional Indian concepts with Western medical science.

Then the Beatles became interested in Transcendental Meditation, under the guidance of the guru Mararishi Mahesh Yogi, who already had a small but committed following in the United States and Europe. Interest in all aspects of

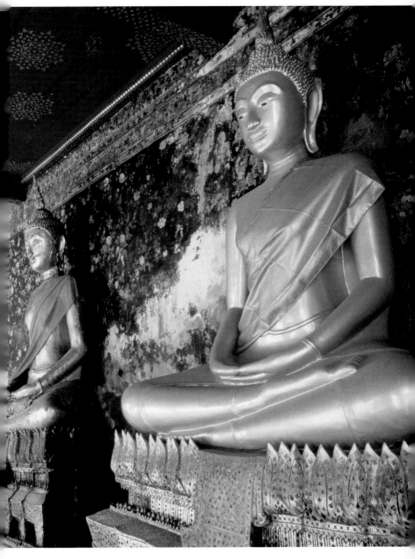

Westerners at long last appreciate the rich cultural heritage of India.

yoga now blossomed in the West. Young people flocked to India, on what would later become known as the "gap year," to discover a philosophy that chimed with the times—non-materialistic, non-egotistical, spiritually enlightening, and with an element of rebellion against the tired old morals and prejudices of their parents.

Coming of Age in the West

So the circle turns—from Western scholars first studying the texts, through a crude fascination with the physical aspects of yoga, followed by the twentieth-century search for meaning, fulfillment, and some kind of answer to a barely articulated question, to today's holistic view. Only now are we beginning to understand what has been known to Eastern sages for centuries.

The rising standard of living in the West made people more health-conscious. They are increasingly aware not just of the importance of diet and exercise, but also of the link between mind and body. Lifestyles, which were once aspired to as being the ultimate achievement, have proved disappointing and the source of yet greater agitation, unhappiness, and ill health. In an age of technological innovation, we work absurdly long, often sedentary hours and suffer for it. Even gaining an end-of-year bonus is, like all blessings, mixed—no matter what we have, there often seems no alternative but to stay on the treadmill to achieve still more. Like Alice in the Lewis Carroll story, we run faster and faster just to stay in the same place.

In the light of this, renewed interest in all aspects of yoga is hardly surprising. It offers what seem to us refreshing and simple ways to step off that treadmill. You will not find it difficult to follow the dietary advice; nor, more importantly, do you have to restrict yourself to one kind of food. As an exercise, yoga is gentle and non-competitive, an asset in a fiercely combative society. Its stretches and poses improve posture, increase flexibility, and tone the system. Just 20 minutes of yoga a day soothes and calms the mind for hours. It encourages healthy sleep, helps to prevent illness, and aids recovery without recourse to drugs.

A disciplined approach to regular practice is recommended, but you can match yoga to your lifestyle and schedule. Young and old, fit and unfit, can all benefit from yoga, provided common-sense guidelines are followed.

However, perhaps the most important aspect of yoga in today's hurly-burly is that it enables those who seek it to find "the space within the heart."

The benefits of practicing yoga draw increasing numbers to classes.

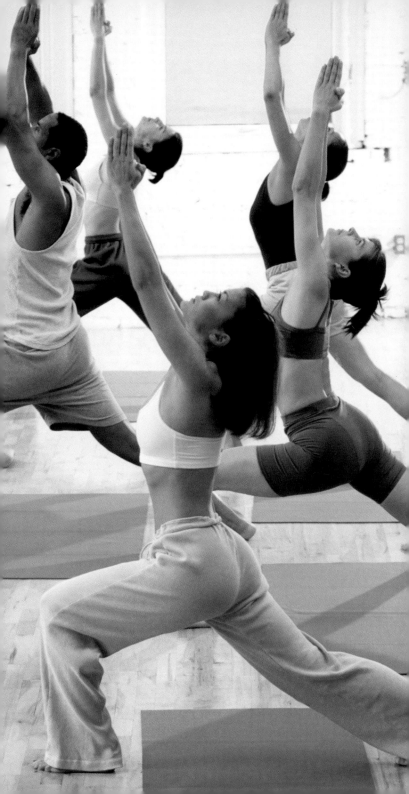

East Meets West

It is not essential to have a detailed grasp of Western human physiology or a full understanding of traditional Ayurvedic medicine in order to benefit from yoga. However, a short survey of both can add an extra dimension to your practice of yoga, helping you focus on what you are doing and avoid the possibility of injury. Questioning fixed ideas by looking at a completely different approach is always healthy.

Your Body

Hatha yoga starts with the body, and what holds the body together is the skeleton. Central to this framework of 206 bones is the spine or backbone. It consists of 33 small bones, called vertebrae, which are separated from each other by a disk of cartilage—firm but flexible tissue, just like that in your outer ear. These are the disks that "slip" when you lift things wrongly. The spine is not straight; it should have three natural curves, but poor posture can put the spine out of alignment, resulting in backache and other discomfort.

The pelvis—hip bones—is a basin-shaped group of bones, pivotal to moving the body and also containing abdominal organs, such as the digestive system. It transfers the weight of the upper body to the legs and feet. Tilting the pelvis too far forward or backward results in poor posture and puts the spine out of alignment. It can also put unnecessary stress on muscles and internal organs. Yoga helps to ensure good posture, and the instruction "tuck in your tail" appears in many of the step-by-step poses in the following chapters.

Bones meet at joints, which are held in place by ligaments. The ends of the bones are protected by cartilage, and the joints are lubricated to make movement easier. The powerhouse of movement is the system of skeletal muscle, which is attached directly or indirectly, via tendons, to the skeleton. These muscles always work in pairs—one contracts while the other relaxes. Both muscles and joints are easily damaged by the abuse we inflict on our own bodies.

A healthy spine is one of the keys to physical well-being.

All organs of the body, of course, have a function, with the possible exception of the appendix. From the point of view of practicing yoga, the two most important internal organs are the lungs and the heart, part of the circulatory system. The lungs are responsible for taking in oxygen and getting rid of carbon dioxide, and their proper function, especially with modern levels of air pollution, is crucial to well-being. Breathing exercises, pranayama, are an important aspect of yoga (*see pages 42–45*). The heart pumps blood around the body, carrying nutrients and oxygen. Heart disease is one of the West's biggest killers, so a healthy heart—and maintaining the correct blood pressure—is literally vital.

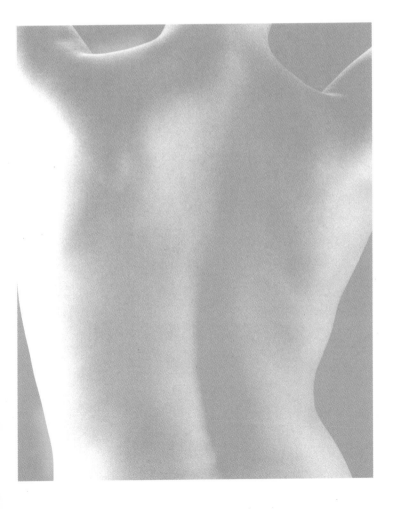

Universal Energy

There are many Eastern philosophies and sciences, such as Taoism and Ayurveda, that view the physiology of the human body in terms of channeling a universal energy. Although the theories are similar, the precise explanation and nomenclature differ. *Prana* is the Sanskrit term for this cosmic energy, which might be described as the total sum of all the energy in the universe.

This energy is channeled through *nadis* to the physical, earthly body. There are said to be some 72,000, each of varying importance. Three in particular are important for the practice of yoga: the *Sushumna* nadi corresponds to the spine, while the *Pingala* nadi flows through the right nostril and the *Ida* nadi through the left nostril. Nadis are located in the astral body—what might be termed the soul—rather than in the physical body. Nevertheless, practicing yoga, especially breathing techniques, helps to keep these astral tubes pure and clear, and maintain the energy balance. If the flow of energy is blocked, illnesses result.

Chakras are the energy centers to which nadis channel prana. The most important seven chakras are located along the Sushumna nidi (*see pages 32–33*). Chakra means wheel, although "vortex" more accurately captures their essence, and each vibrates with its own energy pattern. Each chakra vibrates at a different frequency, from the lowest to the highest, transmitting pranic energy from one level to the next and throughout the physical body. This vibration pattern is associated with a particular color, a letter of the Sanskrit alphabet, a number of lotus petals, and a mantra. If the pattern is incorrect or the flow of energy is either too vigorous or blocked, the result is physical, mental, or emotional imbalance and ill health. Chakras may also close, but this happens only at death.

The concept of balance is central. For example, the Pingala nadi carries sun (*Ha*), male, positive energy, while the Ida nadi carries moon (*Tha*), female, negative energy. As the two nadis intertwine along the length of the Sushumna nadi, carrying pranic energy to the chakras, it is essential that they are in balance. If, for example, the chakra located at the navel is blocking the flow of energy, you may experience feelings of depression, purposelessness, and exhaustion— what in the West would be described as feeling "sick and tired."

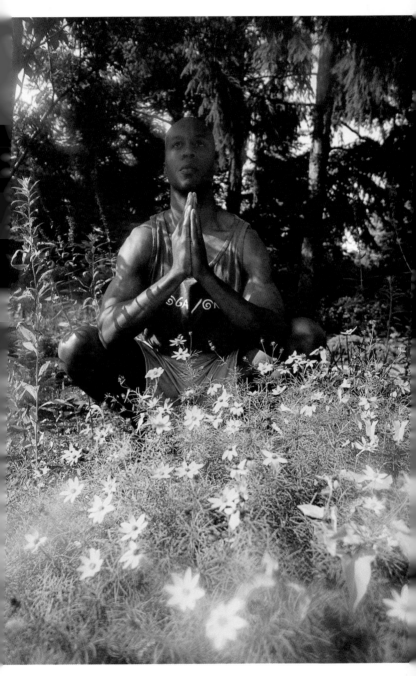

A sense of oneness with everything restores spiritual balance.

The Seven Main Chakras

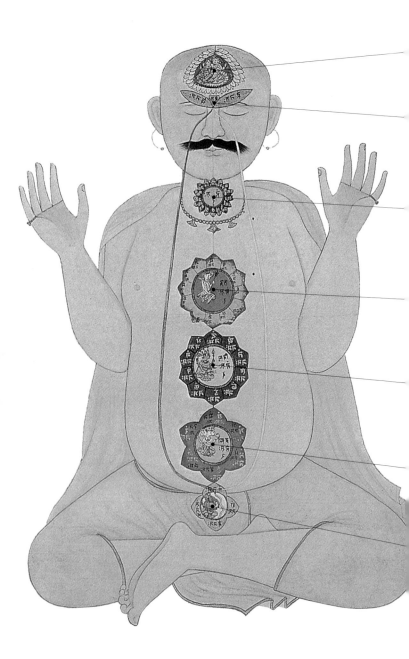

Sahasrara Chakra—Crown Energy Center

Location: top of the head, the cerebrum
Color: ultraviolet
Lotus petals: 1,000
Function: union, wisdom, symbol of the infinite
Physical function: upper brain, pineal gland, pituitary gland
Mantra: Soham

Ajna Chakra—Brow Energy Center

Location: in the middle of the forehead, the "Third Eye"
Color: indigo
Lotus petals: 2
Function: perception, concentration
Physical function: eyes, lower brain, nervous system
Mantra: Om

Vishuddha Chakra—Throat Energy Center

Location: base of the throat
Color: light blue
Lotus petals: 16
Function: creativity, communication
Physical function: thyroid, larynx, ears, respiration, throat
Mantra: Ham

Anahata Chakra—Heart Energy Center

Location: heart
Color: green
Lotus petals: 12
Function: love, including cosmic love
Physical function: heart and circulatory system, lungs, thymus, immune system
Mantra: Yam

Manipura Chakra—Solar Plexus Energy Center

Location: at the navel
Color: yellow
Lotus petals: 10
Function: will, desire, inner sun center
Physical function: digestive system
Mantra: Ram

Swadhishtana Chakra—Sacral Energy Center

Location: genitals
Color: orange
Lotus petals: 6
Function: sexuality, balance
Physical function: reproductive system, bladder, kidneys
Mantra: Vam

Muladhara Chakra—Base or Root Energy Center

Location: perineum (at the base of the spine between the anus and genitals)
Color: red
Lotus petals: 4
Function: grounding, will to live
Physical function: adrenal glands, bowels
Mantra: Lam

What Yoga Can and Cannot Do

The short answer to what yoga can do is that it can help you find your own route to health and vitality, which may include spiritual and emotional as well as physical well-being. It also puts you in touch with yourself. It cannot solve your problems for you, although it can help you compose your mind so that you are more able to find solutions. Equally, it cannot turn back the clock to make you younger, although it can make you look and feel better and fitter, and prevent or alleviate some of the ailments associated with the later years. In this modern age of constant rushing and immediate gratification, it is important to remember that yoga is a path, not an instant answer.

Taking Time

Yoga is non-competitive and requires regular, disciplined practice. If you take up running, you don't expect to break world records the first time you are on the track. Equally, when you take up yoga, don't expect to be able to hold all the poses on the first day. Never force your body into a position that strains it; yoga should not hurt. With daily practice, your muscles and joints will become more flexible and you will gain stamina.

Do not neglect warming-up exercises (*see pages 52–57*). The less fit you are, the more important it is to do them to avoid strain and injury. You don't have to do all of them or do them for very long, but it is sensible to loosen up muscles and joints before you start, especially if you lead a fairly sedentary life. When you are more practiced, you may prefer to warm up with the *Salute to the Sun* (*see page 58*).

Guidelines

It is always sensible to check with your physician before embarking on any exercise program. This is especially important if you have any medical conditions or are convalescing or recovering from an injury (*see pages 36–37*). Yoga can help alleviate many common ailments, including arthritis and backache, but not all poses are advisable. Similarly, check with your physician if you are pregnant, or attend a yoga-for-pregnancy class with a qualified teacher. However, it is not advisable to take up yoga for the first time during pregnancy. Although yoga can be of invaluable assistance in the treatment of many conditions, it is not a substitute for medical care. If you are aware of any symptoms of ill health, consult your physician.

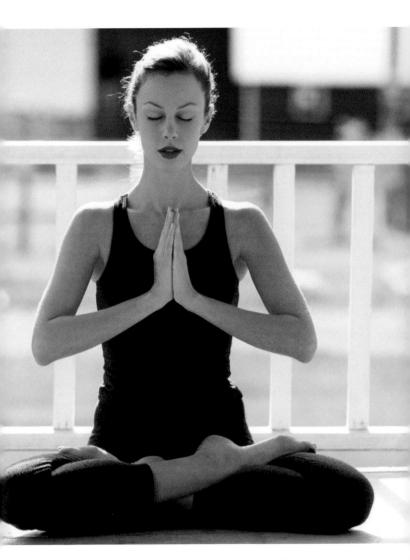

Yoga consists of many paths that can put you in touch with yourself.

Specific Contraindications

- **Asthma** Check with your physician before practicing breathing exercises (pranayama).

- **Back injury** Avoid twists; forward, back, and side bends; and inverted poses, such as head stands and shoulder stands.

- **Breathing problems** Check with your physician before practicing breathing exercises (pranayama).

- **Chronic fatigue syndrome** Check with your physician; avoid standing poses, and proceed very slowly.

- **Dizziness** Avoid inverted poses, such as head stands and shoulder stands; check with your physician before practicing breathing exercises (pranayama).

- **Ear problems** Avoid inverted poses, such as head stands and shoulder stands; check with your physician before practicing breathing exercises (pranayama).

- **Eye problems/injury** Avoid inverted poses, such as head stands and shoulder stands; check with your physician before doing breathing exercises (pranayama).

- **Glaucoma** Avoid inverted poses, such as head stands and shoulder stands.

- **Head injury** Avoid inverted poses, such as head stands and shoulder stands.

- **Heart disease** Avoid standing poses and back bends; check with your physician before practicing breathing exercises (pranayama).

- **High blood pressure** Avoid standing poses; inverted poses, such as head stands and shoulder stands; and back bends.

- **Hip replacement** Avoid sitting poses.

- **Knee injury** Avoid kneeling poses and back bends.

- **Lung problems** Check with your physician before practicing breathing exercises (pranayama).

- **ME** Check with your physician; avoid standing poses and proceed very slowly.

- **Menstruation** Avoid inverted poses, such as head stands and shoulder stands.

- **Migraine** Avoid inverted poses, such as head stands and shoulder stands.

- **Neck injury** Avoid inverted poses, such as head stands and shoulder stands.

- **Osteoporosis** Avoid back bends and inverted poses, such as head stands and shoulder stands, and take extra care with stretches and twists.

- **Pregnancy** Do not take up yoga for the first time during pregnancy; check with your obstetrician if you are already practicing yoga.

- **Sinus problems** Avoid inverted poses, such as head stands and shoulder stands; check with a physician before practicing breathing exercises (pranayama).

- **Slipped (prolapsed) disk** Avoid twists; forward/back bends; and side bends.

WATCHPOINT
Never force your body into a position that causes discomfort, distress, or pain—you can cause injury.

An Emphasis on Purity

The Western saying that "cleanliness is next to Godliness" could equally have originated with the sages of the East, where the purity of the body is emphasized as strongly as that of the mind. A personal hygiene routine, a wholesome diet of natural food, breathing control, and yoga postures have all been devised to cleanse the body in preparation for cleansing the mind.

The Six Cleansing Acts

The *shad kriyas* are techniques for cleansing the body, designed to eliminate toxins and waste products and so prepare the body to achieve maximum benefit from proper breathing and yoga postures. However, they are not widely practiced in the West and some people find them extremely distasteful. It is recommended that anyone interested in learning these techniques should do so with a professional teacher.

- **Dhauti** (stomach cleansing) is designed to remove excess mucus and food particles from the gullet and stomach and consists of swallowing a thin strip of cloth, such as gauze, soaked in warm milk or a weak salt solution.

- **Basti** (colon cleansing) is a method for cleansing the large intestine by drawing water into the bowel while sitting in a tub of water. It is not the same as colonic irrigation or an enema because it controlled by manipulating the abdominal muscles.

- **Neti** (nasal cleansing) helps to cleanse the nasal passage and sinuses. Plain water or a weak salt solution is poured into one nostril by means of a spouted jug and expelled from the other. There are a number of other techniques, such as filling the mouth with water and then expelling it through the nostrils.

Purity of the body is thought to encourage purity of the mind, but it is not essential to follow traditional yoga cleansing techniques.

- **Trataka** (steady gazing) is intended to cleanse the eyes and improve the eyesight. It consists of looking, without blinking, at an object—a lighted candle, for example—placed at eye level and about 28 inches/70 cm away. Trataka is stopped as soon as the eyes start to water.

- **Nauli** (abdominal manipulation) consists of a series of exercises for retracting and rolling or churning the abdominal muscles. It massages the internal organs and helps clear congestion.

- **Kapalabhati** (respiratory cleansing) is designed to cleanse the lungs and invigorate all the body's tissues. It consists of rapidly contracting the abdominal muscles to force air out of the lungs and then relaxing them to let air back in (*see page 45*).

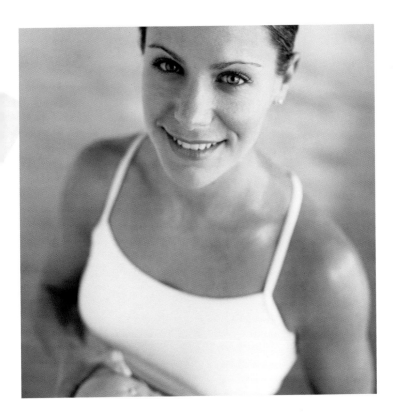

The Pure Diet

The classic texts of yoga divide foods into three categories, as well as recommending some straightforward guidelines about eating. Each of these types of food is thought to influence behavior and health, and individual preferences for certain foods are thought to be a reflection of a person's mental purity and spiritual development.

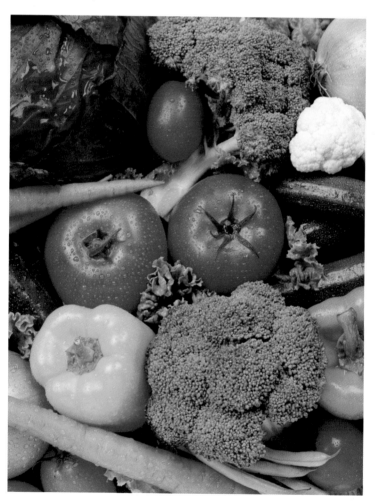

A diet of fresh fruit and vegetables is considered *sattvic* or pure.

- **Sattvic foods** (pure foods) are thought to calm the mind, increase energy, build stamina, and enhance vitality. They include fruit and fruit juice; vegetables, especially salads and raw vegetables; herbs; whole grains; pulses; honey; and dairy products. They should be free of artificial flavorings and preservatives and as fresh as possible.

- **Rajasic foods** (stimulating foods) are sour, salty, bitter, hot, and pungent and are said to overstimulate both the mind and body, causing a restless imbalance and even illnesses, such as circulatory problems. They include onions; garlic; tea; coffee and other caffeine drinks; chocolate; and refined products, such as white flour. Some authorities include meat, fish, eggs, and alcohol in this group. Tobacco products are also said to be *rajasic*.

- **Tamasic foods** (impure foods) are stale, tasteless, fermented, or rotten. Overcooked and burned food and both fried and barbecued dishes are also said to be *tamasic*. Such foods are said to create feelings of lethargy, dullness, and a lack of control that may lead to overeating and ill health. Some people include meat, fish, and eggs in this group. Wine and other fermented alcoholic drinks are said to be tamasic and, nowadays, drugs have been added to the list.

How, as well as what, you eat is also considered important. Simplicity—eating only a few different foods at one meal—is recommended. Moderation avoids overloading the system. Try to leave the table with one-quarter of your stomach still empty. The writers of classical texts advised fasting for one day each week and suggested that you should miss any regular meal if you do not feel hungry at that time. (Before fasting regularly, check with your physician.) Eat in silence or, at least, in tranquillity and chew your food thoroughly. Food is considered a divine gift, so it should be eaten slowly and with enjoyment of its flavor.

While there is much to endorse in yoga's approach to diet, and the emphasis on fresh and unprocessed ingredients is in tune with the World Health Organization's recommendations, it is advisable to avoid making sudden changes to your usual eating habits.

Breathing

Breathing properly is an essential part of learning and practicing yoga postures. People are often surprised to discover that it is not only possible, but common to have spent most of their lives breathing at less than full capacity and without the maximum benefit. After rectifying this, they are also pleasantly surprised to feel improved vitality and energy, with fewer headaches and calmer nerves.

When you are practicing yoga postures or, indeed, in day-to-day life, you should breathe evenly and regularly through the nose. (For some yoga postures, there are specific instructions about breathing.) You should draw air into the lungs by expanding the diaphragm—the large muscle just below the ribcage that separates the chest and abdomen. As air fills the lungs, the muscles between

Try to find a quiet moment each day to sit and breathe rhythmically. Breathe in through your nose to a count of four and then out through your nose for a count of six.

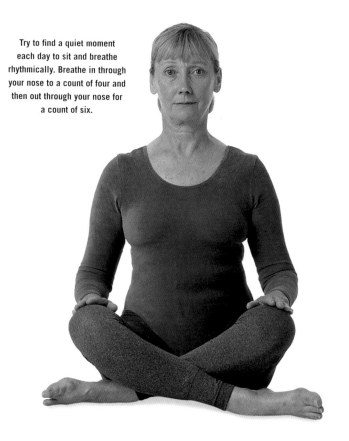

the ribs expand and, finally, air is drawn into the upper part of the chest. This pattern is reversed when you breathe out. Many people fill only part of their lungs with air, starving the blood and organs of the body of the rich supply of oxygen they need.

A Simple Check

To find out if you are using your lungs to their full capacity, try this check.

1 Stand up straight with your shoulders relaxed. Place one hand on your stomach, just below your waist, and the other above it, resting on your ribcage. With your mouth closed, breathe in through your nose, slowly and evenly, feeling your abdomen expand as your diaphragm draws in air. Then you should feel your ribcage expand as the air fills your lungs. Try not to move your shoulders and chest.

2 Breathe out through your nose, slowly and evenly, feeling your abdomen contract, followed by your ribcage. Again, try not to move your chest and shoulders. Do this several times.

Breathing Exercises

Yoga also includes specific breathing exercises, called pranayama. These techniques are designed to channel prana—energy—to the seven main chakras—energy centers (*see pages 32–33*). They help to strengthen and energize the body and also to calm and clear the mind.

WATCHPOINT

Before trying any of the breathing exercises on the following pages, check the list of contraindications on pages 36–37. In general, practicing pranayama is not recommended for people with lung or respiratory disorders, heart problems, blood pressure problems, or serious ear or eye complaints. Pregnant women should check with their obstetricians first. Also, if you start to feel dizzy or tired when doing the exercises, stop immediately. Finally, like all yoga, this is not a competition, so do not try to hold your breath for an inordinately long time.

Anuloma Viloma—Alternate Nostril Breathing

1 Sit cross-legged on the floor with your back straight and your shoulders down. Rest one hand on your knee. Place the index and middle finger of the other hand on the bridge of your nose, so that you can block your nostrils with your thumb and ring finger.

2 Breathe out, then block your right nostril and breathe in through your left nostril to a count of five. Block your left nostril and breathe out through your right nostril to a count of five.

3 Keeping your left nostril blocked, breathe in through your right nostril to a count of five. Block your right nostril and breathe out through your left nostril to a count of five.

These three steps constitute one cycle. Repeat the cycle ten times, concentrating on keeping the rhythm even. If it helps, close your eyes.

A More Advanced Technique

When you have practiced basic alternate nostril breathing, you can add some further steps. Start as in Step 1 above.

1 Breathe out, then block your right nostril and breathe in through your left nostril to a count of five. Block your left nostril as well and hold the breath for a count of ten. Then breathe out through your right nostril to a count of five.

2 Keeping your left nostril blocked, breathe in through your right nostril to a count of five. Block your right nostril as well and hold the breath for a count of ten. Then breathe out through your left nostril to a count of five.

Kapalabhati—Respiratory Cleansing

1 Sit cross-legged on the floor with your shoulders relaxed, your mouth closed, and your hands resting on your knees. Breathe in, then sharply contract your abdominal muscles to force the air out of your lungs through your nostrils.

2 Immediately relax your abdominal muscles to let air enter your lungs, keeping your mouth closed.

3 Repeat these two steps nine more times in quick succession. Breathe slowly and evenly three times, then repeat. Do not continue this exercise for more than one minute in each session.

Breath Retention

1 Sit cross-legged on the floor with your shoulders relaxed, your mouth closed, and your hands resting on your knees. Breathe out through your nose, then breathe in to a count of four. Hold your breath for a count of four. Exhale.

2 Breathe in again to a count of four, then hold your breath for a count of four. Breathe in again, then hold your breath for a count of four.

3 Breathe out through your nose slowly and completely. Repeat twice more, then relax.

Getting Started

You can practice yoga almost anywhere—indoors or outdoors. In fact, you can use some of the techniques and exercises to relieve stress at the office desk or to ease tired muscles and boost the circulation on a long car journey. However, to help ensure that yoga is incorporated regularly into your daily routine and to benefit fully from it, it is useful to have a designated "yoga space" that is free from distractions. This doesn't need to be huge, but do make sure that you have plenty of room to stretch without banging into furniture or breaking ornaments. It should also be well ventilated and neither freezing cold nor stiflingly hot.

You will need a level floor for all the postures, whether standing, sitting, kneeling, or lying down. A bed is far too soft and yielding, and you risk falling off and injuring yourself. You can buy yoga mats to provide some cushioning, but a folded blanket serves the purpose just as well. A small cushion may provide beginners with extra support for seated poses.

What Should You Wear?

You don't have to buy expensive exercise clothes and some people find loose, baggy garments the most comfortable. So long as your clothes do not restrict movement or make it difficult to breathe, you can wear anything you like. You can even practice the postures stark naked in the privacy of your own home, if that suits you. Although yoga is a very gentle form of exercise, you can work up a sweat, so lightweight, natural fabrics may be the best choice. Don't wear anything on your feet, as you need direct contact with the ground. This not only helps exercise all the joints of the ankles and toes and improve their strength and flexibility, but it will help you feel grounded.

**You do not require special clothes or equipment to practice yoga—
just a quiet place where you won't be distracted.**

First Things First

Yoga postures and a full stomach are not compatible, so try to schedule your regular sessions at least two, preferably three hours after a main meal or one hour after a light snack. Many people find that first thing in the morning is the ideal time, especially as they benefit from the session throughout the rest of the day. Empty your bladder and, if possible, your bowels, and clear your nose so that you can breathe easily.

Start with one of the relaxation postures (*see pages 50–51*), then do some warming-up exercises (*see pages 52–57*), relaxing in between. Never force your body beyond its capacity or strain to achieve a posture. Concentrate fully on each posture and return gently rather than jerkily to your starting position. Relax in between. Enjoy your yoga session.

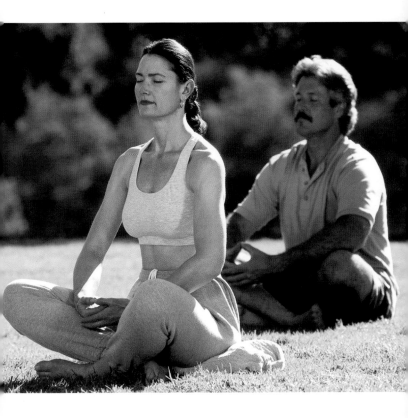

How Long Is a Session?

It is well known that if you want to find time to do something, you will, however busy your life, and this is a good reason for setting aside a regular schedule. Most yoga classes take between 1½ and 2 hours. At home, an hour a day is ideal, but if you can't manage this, even 30 minutes is beneficial. Anything less than 20 minutes will rush things too much. If you can't find time to schedule a daily session, try to manage two or three sessions spread out over the week.

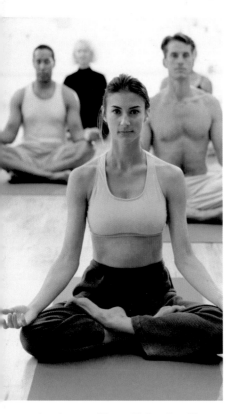

Learning yoga with a qualified teacher will ensure that you understand the poses correctly and do not injure yourself.

Teachers and Classes

The best way to start learning about yoga is under the guidance of a professional teacher. There are many centers that provide classes or that can put you in touch with a qualified teacher (*see page 204*). Of course, if you go to a class, you can still practice at home on the other days of the week. There are also tapes and videos available.

If you are going to learn from a book, you might find it helpful to record the steps of each position on to a tape. This is easier than craning to look at the next instruction or stopping and starting, which can disturb not only your concentration, but also your balance. Working alternately with a friend reading out loud is another helpful way of learning new positions.

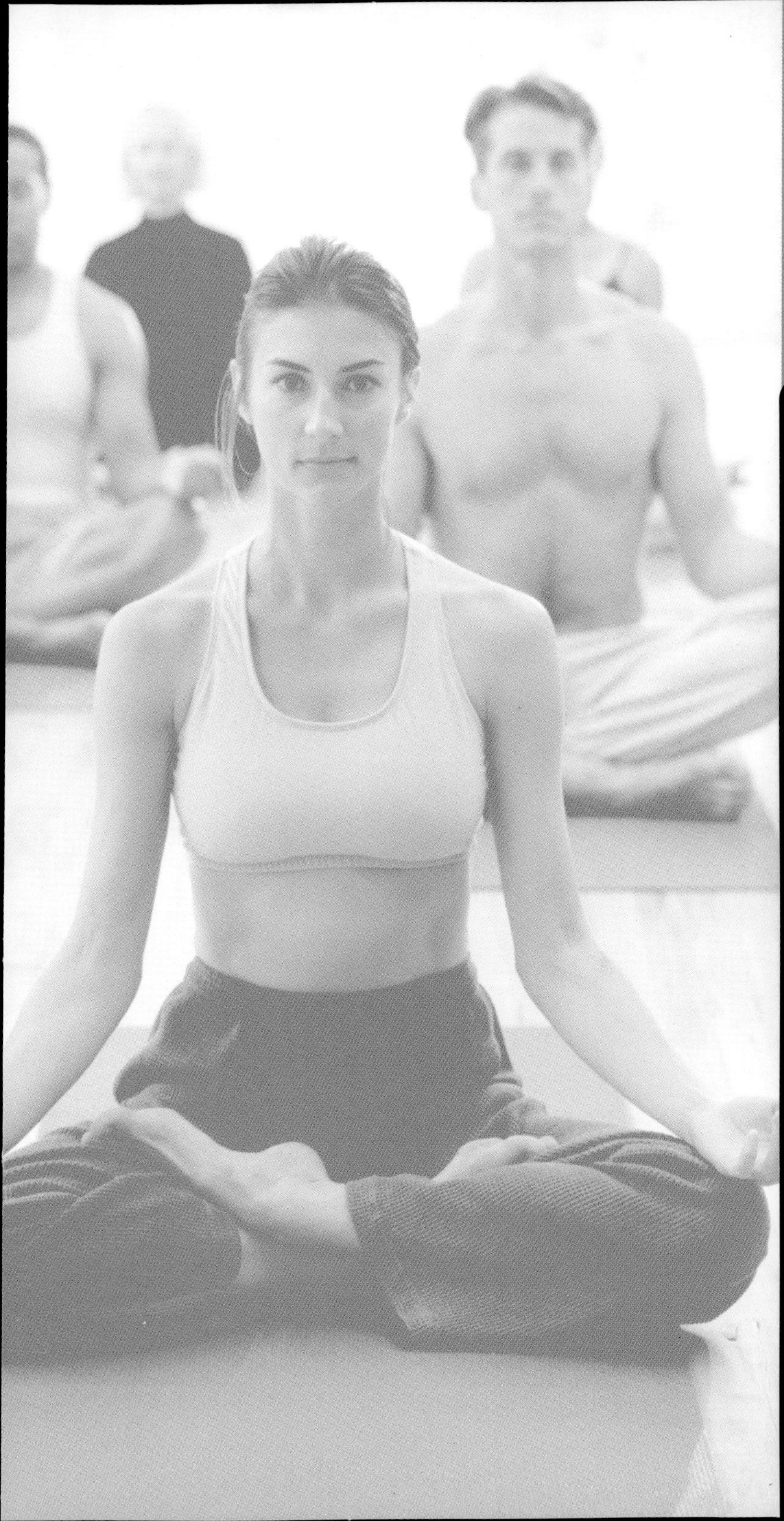

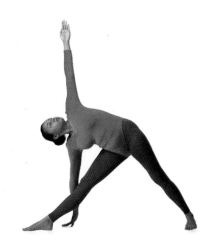

Learning Poses

The *Gheranda Samhita* states that there are "eighty-four hundreds of thousands" of asanas, or postures. Hatha yoga incorporates rather fewer, but includes a wide range of poses, some of which require a lifetime's experience. However, there are many less demanding positions, requiring only a basic level of fitness. The exercises and positions described in this chapter, if learned and practiced properly in a well-balanced program (*see pages 50–100*), will start you on a gentle route to becoming more fit, supple, and relaxed. Some may seem almost childishly simple, so you may be surprised at how much concentration and practice are needed to get them absolutely right.

The Importance of Posture

The ways in which we stand, sit, and even lie in bed affect every aspect of our health and well-being. Unfortunately, bad habits—slumping in front of the television at the end of a busy day, for example—are all too easy to acquire. Fortunately, good (even perfect) posture can be learned and, if maintained, can reverse many problems acquired through bad posture. Proper posture is not only vital to our everyday well-being, it is also the essential starting point for any yoga position. Standing, sitting, and kneeling are common starting positions for many poses in this chapter.

Easy Position

Called *Sukasana*, this is the starting point for sitting positions. With practice, your knees will gradually lower until they rest comfortably on the floor. Beginners may find it helpful to sit on a small cushion.

Sit cross-legged on the floor, resting your hands lightly on your knees or cupped in your lap—do not clasp them. The classic *Chin Mudra* position for the hands is to rest the backs of them on your knees and bring the tips of the thumbs and index fingers together. Straighten and lift your spine so that it is in line with your neck and head. Breathe naturally through your nose. You should feel centered and relaxed. Practice the *Easy position* with both right over left and left over right ankles.

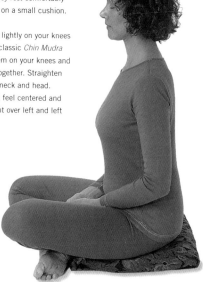

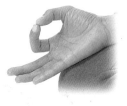

The classic *Chin Mudra* position

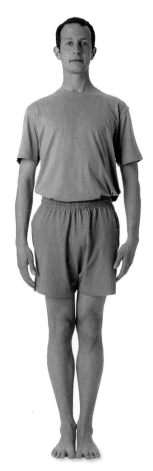

PRACTICE MAKES PERFECT

To begin with, it may help to practice in front of a mirror—sideways on in the case of the *Upright Steadiness*—to ensure that you are in the correct position. Better still, ask a friend to observe critically or take Polaroid photographs.

Practice all these positions regularly for several minutes each day. If your knees are a bit creaky, maintain the *Classic Thunderbolt* posture for at least one minute, then bounce gently up and down a few times to loosen the ligaments.

Upright Steadiness

Most standing positions start from this posture and it is worth adopting it routinely whenever you are standing. Upright Steadiness is a literal translation of the Sanskrit word *Samasthiti,* but the position is also known as *Tadasana,* the Mountain.

Stand with your feet together, with your weight evenly balanced over the full length of both feet, and your arms by your sides. Hold your head erect with your chin level and keep your shoulders down. This should result in your chest lifting naturally—do not thrust it forward. Tuck in your tummy and the base of your spine. You should feel centered and poised.

The Classic Thunderbolt

With the Sanskrit name *Vajrasana,* this pose is known by a variety of English names, including the Diamond. This kneeling position comes less easily to Westerners and will require frequent, although not necessarily prolonged, practice.

Kneel, sitting back on your heels and keeping the tops of your feet and your toes flat on the floor. Spread your heels slightly apart so that their inner edges support the outer edges of your bottom, but keep toes and knees together. Rest your hands, palms downward, lightly on your knees. Raise your spine so that head, neck, and spine are in alignment, then straighten your elbows. Breathe naturally through your nose.

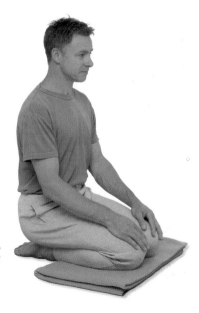

Warming Up

Stretches

All exercise, no matter how gentle, should be preceded by
a warm-up routine to avoid injury, and yoga is no exception.
This is particularly important for beginners. *The Salute to the Sun*
(*see pages 58–59*) is the traditional warm-up because it tones all
the body's muscles and releases tension in the spine. However,
beginners may prefer to use some more familiar exercise
routines until they feel more confident.

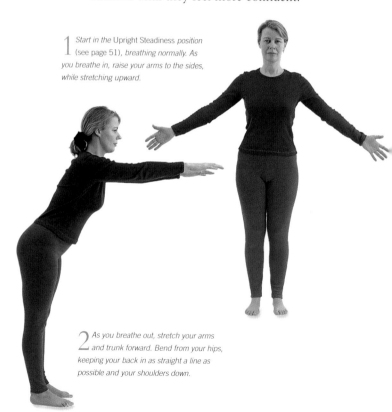

1 *Start in the* Upright Steadiness *position
(see page 51), breathing normally. As
you breathe in, raise your arms to the sides,
while stretching upward.*

2 *As you breathe out, stretch your arms
and trunk forward. Bend from your hips,
keeping your back in as straight a line as
possible and your shoulders down.*

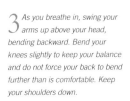

3 *As you breathe in, swing your arms up above your head, bending backward. Bend your knees slightly to keep your balance and do not force your back to bend further than is comfortable. Keep your shoulders down.*

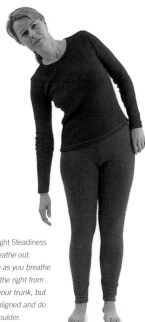

4 *Return to the Upright Steadiness position as you breathe out. Breathe normally, then as you breathe out, bend sideways to the right from the hips. Do not twist your trunk, but try to keep your body aligned and do not hunch your left shoulder.*

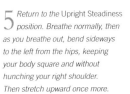

5 *Return to the Upright Steadiness position. Breathe normally, then as you breathe out, bend sideways to the left from the hips, keeping your body square and without hunching your right shoulder. Then stretch upward once more.*

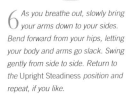

6 *As you breathe out, slowly bring your arms down to your sides. Bend forward from your hips, letting your body and arms go slack. Swing gently from side to side. Return to the Upright Steadiness position and repeat, if you like.*

Head and Neck Rolls

Balance is an important aspect of yoga—a forward bend,

for example, should be balanced by a back bend. You should

therefore follow this sequence twice, turning first to the

left and then to the right.

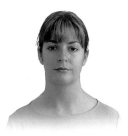

1 *Start in the* Upright Steadiness, Easy, *or* Classic
Thunderbolt *position (see pages 50–51),
whichever is most comfortable. As you breathe in,
imagine that a string is attached to your head and
lifting it straight toward the ceiling. Keep your
shoulders down and relaxed.*

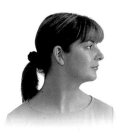

2 *As you breathe out, gently turn your head
to the left. Holding the position, breathe in.
Then, as you breathe out, try to turn your head
slightly further to the left, without straining your
neck. Holding the position, breathe in.*

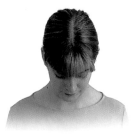

3 *As you breathe out, gently roll your head
downward to rest your chin on your chest.
Keep your spine straight and breathe normally,
gently lowering your head with each out breath.*

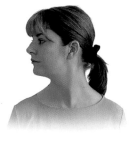

4 *As you breathe in, gently roll your head up and
round to the right, keeping your shoulders
level. Holding the position, breathe in. Then, as you
breathe out, try to turn your head slightly further to
the right, without straining your neck. Holding the
position, breathe in. Breathe out and return to face
the front. Repeat the sequence, clockwise this time.*

Shoulder Shrugging

This exercise not only loosens up the shoulders before the poses, but is also a good way of relieving tension, which often causes stiffness to the muscles in the shoulders and upper back.

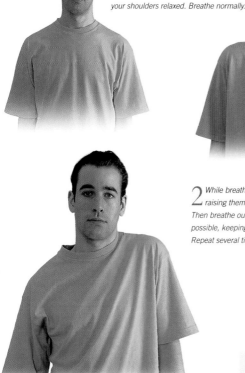

1 *Start in the* Upright Steadiness, Easy, *or* Classic Thunderbolt *position* (see pages 50–51), *whichever is most comfortable. Keep your head straight and your shoulders relaxed. Breathe normally.*

2 *While breathing in, shrug both your shoulders, raising them as close to your ears as you can. Then breathe out and flop them down as low as possible, keeping your spine straight throughout. Repeat several times.*

3 *While breathing in, shrug your left shoulder only, keeping the right one relaxed. Then breathe out and flop it down as low as possible, keeping your spine straight throughout. Repeat, shrugging your right shoulder only. Repeat the whole step several times.*

SHOULDER ROLLS

Place your hands on your shoulders. Breathe normally, gently rolling your shoulders in the largest circles you can six times. Then stop and roll them six times in the opposite direction.

Arms and Finger Joints

Stretching the arms and flexing the fingers improves the
circulation and loosens the joints. These exercises are also
beneficial to anyone who spends a lot of time at a computer
keyboard. Done regularly, they can help prevent repetitive strain
injury (RSI). You can do them sitting at your desk.

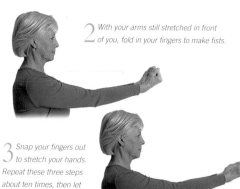

2 With your arms still stretched in front
of you, fold in your fingers to make fists.

1 Start in the Upright
Steadiness or Easy position
(see pages 50–51) or sit up
straight on a chair or stool.
Breathing normally, stretch out
your arms in front of you, palms
upward. Then bend your elbows
and place your fingertips on
your shoulders. As you breathe
out, fling your arms forward.

3 Snap your fingers out
to stretch your hands.
Repeat these three steps
about ten times, then let
your hands go limp and
shake them from the wrists.

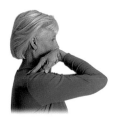

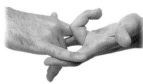

4 Hold your hands level with your chest,
palms downward and with the tips of the
middle fingers just touching, then turn your
left hand palm upward. Stretch the index
and little fingers of both hands out to the
sides. Bend the two middle fingers of your
left hand up and the two middle fingers of
your right hand down. Move your hands
closer together, sliding your right index finger
over your left little finger and your right little
finger over your left index finger.

5 Turn your left hand
toward you and
straighten the two middle
fingers so that they are
lying across the knuckle
of your right index finger.
Raise your right thumb
and press it down on the
tip of the two middle
fingers. Open your palms.

6 Straighten your two
right middle fingers
away from you, then tuck
your left thumb beneath
the tips. You may need to
move your hands further
apart. Do not tense your
shoulders when doing this
finger twist and don't force
your fingers if they are
becoming painful.

Leg and Toe Joints

Feet really take a beating every day, so it's a good idea to
kick off your shoes and give your toes and ankles some attention.
At the same time, you can stretch the hamstrings, those
tendons at the back of the knee.

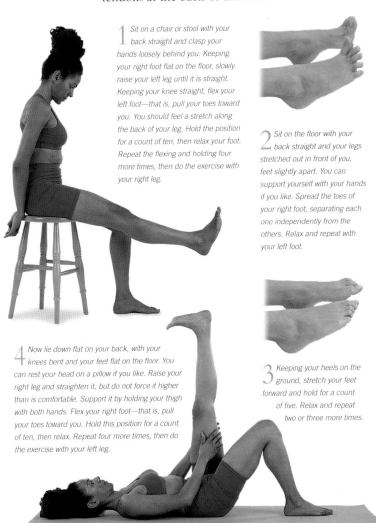

1 Sit on a chair or stool with your back straight and clasp your hands loosely behind you. Keeping your right foot flat on the floor, slowly raise your left leg until it is straight. Keeping your knee straight, flex your left foot—that is, pull your toes toward you. You should feel a stretch along the back of your leg. Hold the position for a count of ten, then relax your foot. Repeat the flexing and holding four more times, then do the exercise with your right leg.

2 Sit on the floor with your back straight and your legs stretched out in front of you, feet slightly apart. You can support yourself with your hands if you like. Spread the toes of your right foot, separating each one independently from the others. Relax and repeat with your left foot.

3 Keeping your heels on the ground, stretch your feet forward and hold for a count of five. Relax and repeat two or three more times.

4 Now lie down flat on your back, with your knees bent and your feet flat on the floor. You can rest your head on a pillow if you like. Raise your right leg and straighten it, but do not force it higher than is comfortable. Support it by holding your thigh with both hands. Flex your right foot—that is, pull your toes toward you. Hold this position for a count of ten, then relax. Repeat four more times, then do the exercise with your left leg.

The Salute to the Sun

Surya Namaskar is not a single pose, but a series of movements synchronized with your breathing. Learn it in stages: each step comprises a single movement, and the right breathing is critical. With practice, it will become rhythmic, free-flowing, and fast—experienced practitioners complete it within about 20 seconds.

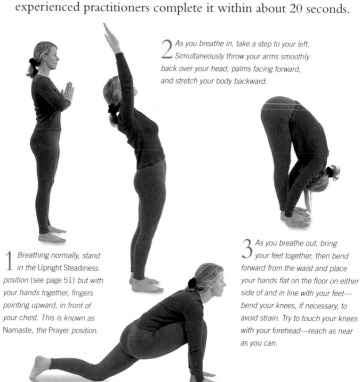

2 As you breathe in, take a step to your left. Simultaneously throw your arms smoothly back over your head, palms facing forward, and stretch your body backward.

1 Breathing normally, stand in the Upright Steadiness position (see page 51) but with your hands together, fingers pointing upward, in front of your chest. This is known as Namaste, the Prayer position.

3 As you breathe out, bring your feet together, then bend forward from the waist and place your hands flat on the floor on either side of and in line with your feet—bend your knees, if necessary, to avoid strain. Try to touch your knees with your forehead—reach as near as you can.

4 Keeping your hands in place and breathing in, take your left leg back as far as you can, bending your toes to grip the floor. Then lower your right knee and raise your head.

5 Holding your breath and without moving your hands, straighten your left leg and take your right leg back to line up with it, while straightening your arms so that you end up supported on your hands and toes, as at the end of a push-up. Keep your head up.

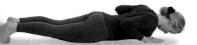

6 While breathing out, lower your knees, then bend your arms and lower your chest and forehead to the floor. Keep your abdominal muscles firm to prevent your tummy from touching the floor.

7 Breathing in, stretch your feet back and straighten your arms, raising your head, shoulders, and chest from the floor and looking upward. (This is the Cobra, see pages 78–79.) There should be no tension in your neck and shoulders.

8 While breathing out, contract your abdominal muscles and raise your hips. Then lower your toes and heels flat to the floor if you can, but do not strain. Simultaneously, swing your head down in between your straightened arms.

9 While breathing in, bring your left leg forward so that your left foot is in between and in line with your hands, and stretch your head up. Simultaneously, lower your right knee to the floor.

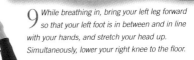

10 While breathing out, bring your left foot forward to align with the right. Without moving your hands, straighten your legs as much as you can. Touch your knees with your forehead as nearly as you can. (This is the same position as Step 3.)

11 While breathing in, take a step to the right. Then straighten up your body, throwing your arms smoothly back over your head, palms facing forward, and stretch your body backward. (This is the same position as Step 2.)

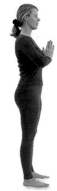

12 While breathing out, bring your feet together and your hands into the Prayer position. Repeat the entire sequence, substituting left for right and vice versa.

The Corpse

It is important to relax between asanas and at the end of a yoga session. The best-known and most restful position for this is *Savasana*, the Corpse or Complete Rest Position.

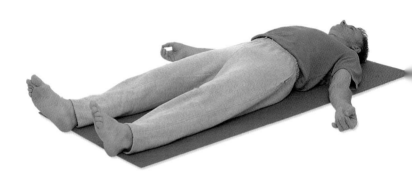

Lie flat on your back with your hands at your sides, palms upward and with the fingers limp and lightly curled. If this feels uncomfortable, you can place your hands palms down and flat on the floor. Stretch out your legs, although not rigidly, with your feet slightly apart, letting them flop slightly sideways. Breathe deeply for one to two minutes. Close your eyes and concentrate on each muscle group in turn, "letting go" of each part of the body. Inhale, tightening the chosen muscles. Hold for a count of five, then exhale and release. When you are completely relaxed, breathe deeply for at least five minutes more without otherwise moving. When you have finished, roll gently on to your side and get up slowly.

RELAXATION SEQUENCE

1	right foot	10	chest	19	left shoulder
2	right calf	11	upper back	20	throat
3	right thigh	12	right hand	21	neck
4	left foot	13	right forearm	22	jaw
5	left calf	14	right upper arm	23	mouth
6	left thigh	15	right shoulder	24	eyes
7	bottom	16	left hand	25	forehead
8	tummy	17	left forearm	26	scalp
9	lower back	18	left upper arm		

Rescue Pose

Westerners are not used to lying on the ground, but it is worth persevering: this position may be used for resting after yoga, and is also a good one for sleeping, because it does not interfere with the circulation. It is particularly beneficial to people with back problems and pregnant women. Lie on your right or left side.

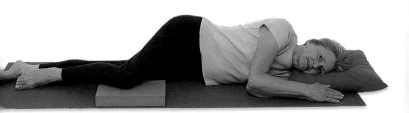

Rest your head on a cushion or pillow so that your head, neck, and spine are in line. If you are on your left side with your left cheek on the cushion, bend your left leg slightly and bring your right knee over to rest on the floor. Bend your elbows and rest your right hand and forearm on top of your left hand and forearm (as shown).
Alternatively, extend your left arm in front of you, palm upward, and let your right arm dangle across your diaphragm. Breathe normally.

THE CROCODILE

This prone posture is good for relaxing, but is not suitable for sleeping because it will restrict breathing. Lie on the floor, face down with your chin resting on the floor. Extend your arms in front of you with the palm of one hand resting on the back of the other. Keep your legs together, pointing your toes. Breathe normally.

The Child

This is a good posture for relaxing if you find lying on your back uncomfortable, and is especially useful after backward stretches. It stimulates the blood flow to the face, scalp, and brain and so has a re-energizing effect. There are a number of variations.

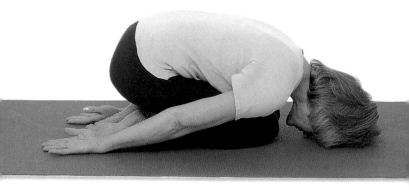

The Child Pose

Start in the *Classic Thunderbolt (see page 51)* and breathe in. While breathing out, gently lower your forehead, rounding your back, until your forehead is touching the floor in front of your knees. At the same time, take your arms back, palms upward, so the backs of your fingers are touching the floor beside your feet. Breathing normally, hold for a count of five, then inhale and slowly return to the *Classic Thunderbolt*.

WATCHPOINT
Not suitable for people with high blood pressure or heart problems.

Variation of the Child

Sometimes called the *Salaam* posture, this is a variation of the Child. As before, start in the *Classic Thunderbolt*. Breathe in and raise your arms straight up, palms facing forward. While breathing out, lower your arms forward, while gently lowering your forehead and rounding your back, until your forehead is touching the floor in front of your knees and your palms are flat on the floor in front of you. Breathing normally, hold for a count of five, then inhale and slowly raise your arms and body upright. Lower your hands to your knees to return to the *Classic Thunderbolt*.

The Hare

The legs, feet, back, shoulders, and neck are all released by this posture, which, like the Child, increases the flow of blood to the brain, face, and scalp. It also allows the pelvis to gently open and release the lower back. It is a useful preparation for inverted postures, such as the Headstand.

1 *Start in a kneeling position with your head, neck, and spine in line. Your toes should be touching and your knees should be a comfortable distance apart so that your lower legs make a V-shape. Lower your bottom on to your upturned heels and place your elbows on the floor beneath your shoulders, with your forearms flat and your fingers pointing forward.*

2 *As you breathe out, gently lower your head so that your forehead rests on the floor, but do not raise your hips. Breathing normally, hold the position for a count of five, then as you breathe in, gently return to your original kneeling position.*

WATCHPOINT

Not suitable for people with high blood pressure or heart problems. Do not stand up quickly when you have finished.

THE EMBARRASSED CHILD

This is similar to the *Hare*. Kneel on the floor with your back and thighs in line. Interlock your fingers and cup the back of your head in your palms. As you breathe out, gently lower the top of your head, not your forehead, to the floor, rounding your back. Rest your forearms and the sides of your hands on the floor and keep your elbows beneath your shoulders. Breathing normally, hold this position for a count of five. Then, as you breathe in, gently return to your original kneeling position.

The Warrior

There are a number of versions of *Virabhadrasana*, the
Warrior, but they all help to strengthen the legs and hips,
stretch the upper body and arms, and are said to increase
vigor and stimulate the system.

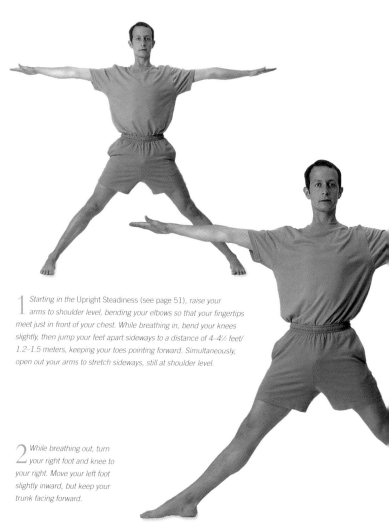

1 *Starting in the* Upright Steadiness *(see page 51), raise your
arms to shoulder level, bending your elbows so that your fingertips
meet just in front of your chest. While breathing in, bend your knees
slightly, then jump your feet apart sideways to a distance of 4–4½ feet/
1.2–1.5 meters, keeping your toes pointing forward. Simultaneously,
open out your arms to stretch sideways, still at shoulder level.*

2 *While breathing out, turn
your right foot and knee to
your right. Move your left foot
slightly inward, but keep your
trunk facing forward.*

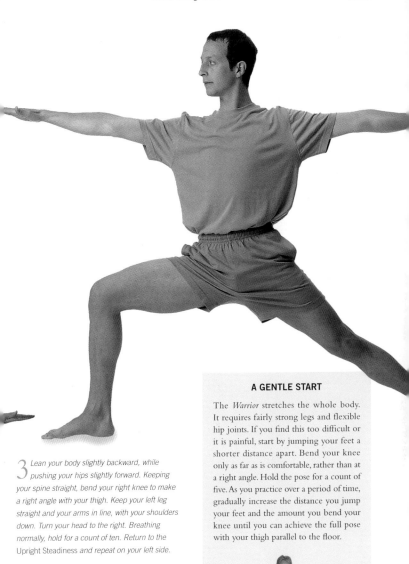

3 Lean your body slightly backward, while pushing your hips slightly forward. Keeping your spine straight, bend your right knee to make a right angle with your thigh. Keep your left leg straight and your arms in line, with your shoulders down. Turn your head to the right. Breathing normally, hold for a count of ten. Return to the Upright Steadiness and repeat on your left side.

A GENTLE START

The *Warrior* stretches the whole body. It requires fairly strong legs and flexible hip joints. If you find this too difficult or it is painful, start by jumping your feet a shorter distance apart. Bend your knee only as far as is comfortable, rather than at a right angle. Hold the pose for a count of five. As you practice over a period of time, gradually increase the distance you jump your feet and the amount you bend your knee until you can achieve the full pose with your thigh parallel to the floor.

The Tree

This posture, *Vrksasana*, improves balance and concentration and also helps to strengthen the ankles and tone the leg muscles. Learn the pose in easy stages without forcing your legs into positions that are uncomfortable. Gradually increase the time you hold the pose to a count of 30.

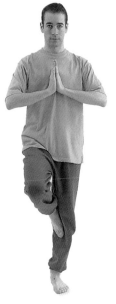

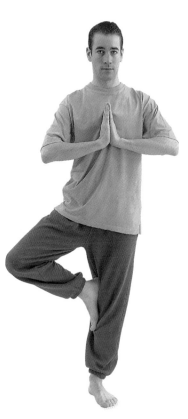

1 *Start in the* Upright Steadiness *(see page 51). Place the sole of your right foot on your left knee and gently swing your right knee backward and outward, but do not force it into an uncomfortable position. Pressing back with your left leg and stretching the muscle just above your kneecap will help brace your supporting leg, but make sure that you keep your hips square. Grip the floor with the toes of your left foot to prevent it from wobbling. When you are balanced and still, breathe in and place your hands in the* Prayer *position. Hold the position for a count of five, breathing normally. Return to the* Upright Steadiness *and repeat standing on your right leg.*

2 *Each time you practice this, try to swing your knee further back and out until it is pointing to the side, but make sure your hips are square. Increase the length of time you hold the pose to at least a count of ten. As you practice, gradually place the sole of your foot higher up your leg.*

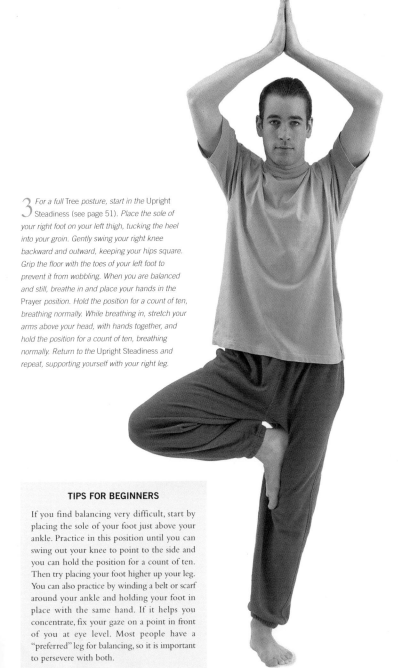

3 *For a full* Tree *posture, start in the* Upright Steadiness *(see page 51).* Place the sole of your right foot on your left thigh, tucking the heel into your groin. Gently swing your right knee backward and outward, keeping your hips square. Grip the floor with the toes of your left foot to prevent it from wobbling. When you are balanced and still, breathe in and place your hands in the Prayer *position. Hold the position for a count of ten, breathing normally. While breathing in, stretch your arms above your head, with hands together, and hold the position for a count of ten, breathing normally. Return to the* Upright Steadiness *and repeat, supporting yourself with your right leg.*

TIPS FOR BEGINNERS

If you find balancing very difficult, start by placing the sole of your foot just above your ankle. Practice in this position until you can swing out your knee to point to the side and you can hold the position for a count of ten. Then try placing your foot higher up your leg. You can also practice by winding a belt or scarf around your ankle and holding your foot in place with the same hand. If it helps you concentrate, fix your gaze on a point in front of you at eye level. Most people have a "preferred" leg for balancing, so it is important to persevere with both.

The Eagle

Garudasana, or the Eagle, improves balance, concentration, and coordination; strengthens the knees, ankles, and calf muscles; and enhances the flexibility of the shoulders. It helps to tone the thighs and is said to eliminate cellulite.

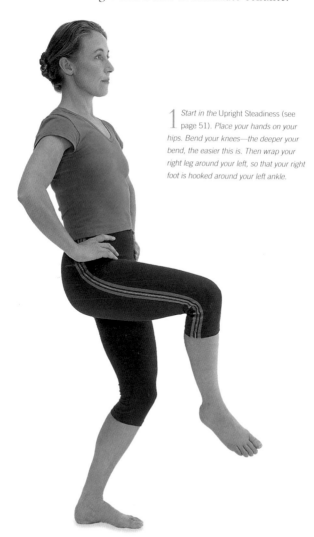

1 *Start in the* Upright Steadiness *(see page 51). Place your hands on your hips. Bend your knees—the deeper your bend, the easier this is. Then wrap your right leg around your left, so that your right foot is hooked around your left ankle.*

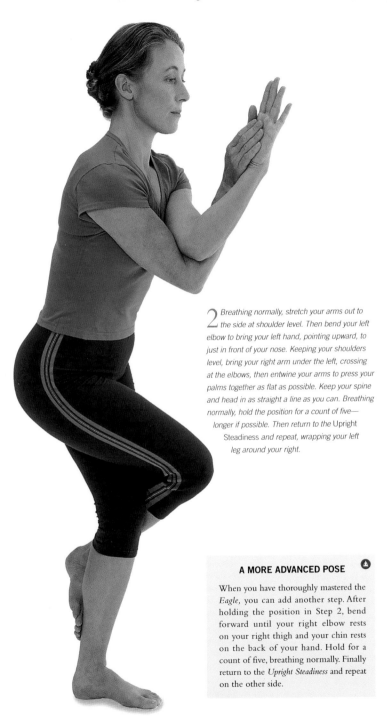

2 Breathing normally, stretch your arms out to the side at shoulder level. Then bend your left elbow to bring your left hand, pointing upward, to just in front of your nose. Keeping your shoulders level, bring your right arm under the left, crossing at the elbows, then entwine your arms to press your palms together as flat as possible. Keep your spine and head in as straight a line as you can. Breathing normally, hold the position for a count of five—longer if possible. Then return to the Upright Steadiness and repeat, wrapping your left leg around your right.

A MORE ADVANCED POSE

When you have thoroughly mastered the *Eagle*, you can add another step. After holding the position in Step 2, bend forward until your right elbow rests on your right thigh and your chin rests on the back of your hand. Hold for a count of five, breathing normally. Finally return to the *Upright Steadiness* and repeat on the other side.

The Triangle

Trikonasana, the Triangle, stretches the body; strengthens and tones the leg muscles; improves the flexibility of the hips; and gets rid of superfluous fat accumulated around the waistline.

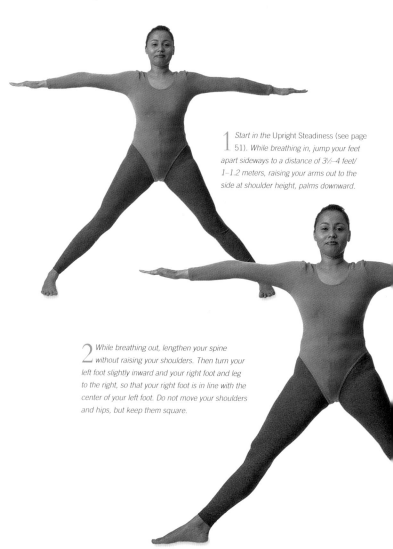

1 *Start in the* Upright Steadiness *(see page 51). While breathing in, jump your feet apart sideways to a distance of 3½–4 feet/ 1–1.2 meters, raising your arms out to the side at shoulder height, palms downward.*

2 *While breathing out, lengthen your spine without raising your shoulders. Then turn your left foot slightly inward and your right foot and leg to the right, so that your right foot is in line with the center of your left foot. Do not move your shoulders and hips, but keep them square.*

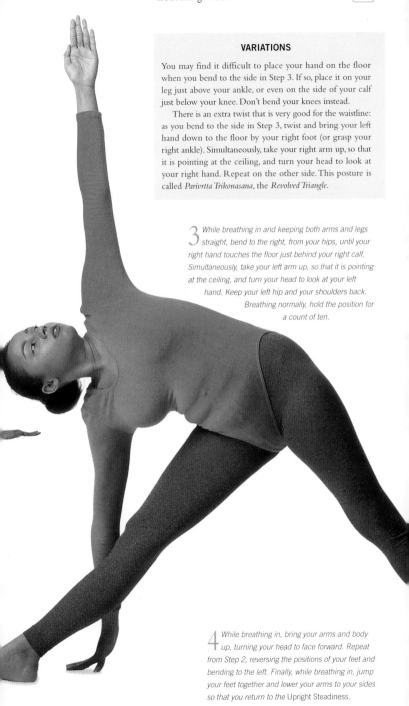

VARIATIONS

You may find it difficult to place your hand on the floor when you bend to the side in Step 3. If so, place it on your leg just above your ankle, or even on the side of your calf just below your knee. Don't bend your knees instead.

There is an extra twist that is very good for the waistline: as you bend to the side in Step 3, twist and bring your left hand down to the floor by your right foot (or grasp your right ankle). Simultaneously, take your right arm up, so that it is pointing at the ceiling, and turn your head to look at your right hand. Repeat on the other side. This posture is called *Parivrtta Trikonasana*, the *Revolved Triangle*.

3 While breathing in and keeping both arms and legs straight, bend to the right, from your hips, until your right hand touches the floor just behind your right calf. Simultaneously, take your left arm up, so that it is pointing at the ceiling, and turn your head to look at your left hand. Keep your left hip and your shoulders back. Breathing normally, hold the position for a count of ten.

4 While breathing in, bring your arms and body up, turning your head to face forward. Repeat from Step 2, reversing the positions of your feet and bending to the left. Finally, while breathing in, jump your feet together and lower your arms to your sides so that you return to the Upright Steadiness.

The Cat

This spinal stretch mimics the action of that most supple and graceful of creatures, the cat. It improves the flexibility of the spine and eases tension in the neck and shoulders. It aids digestion and circulation, and can relieve constipation and period pains. It is also usually included in postnatal yoga classes.

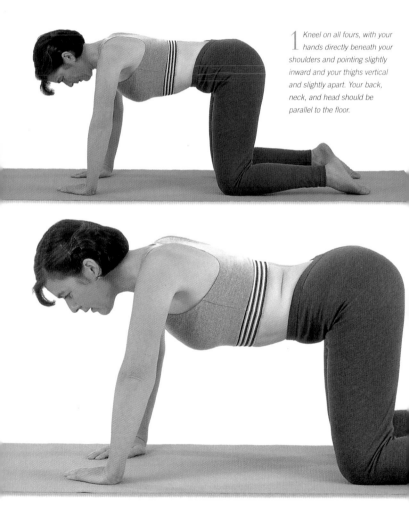

1 *Kneel on all fours, with your hands directly beneath your shoulders and pointing slightly inward and your thighs vertical and slightly apart. Your back, neck, and head should be parallel to the floor.*

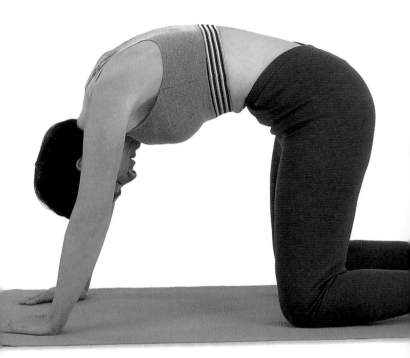

2 While breathing in, tense your abdominal muscles and hollow your spine, lowering the trunk between shoulders and hips as far as possible without bending your arms. Simultaneously, lift your head up and back. Hold the position for a count of ten, breathing normally.

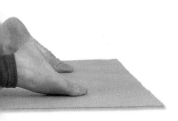

3 In a single smooth movement and while breathing out, arch your back, raising your spine as high as you can and lowering your head between your arms. Don't bend your arms and try to avoid pushing up from your elbows. Hold the position for a count of ten, breathing normally. Repeat several times.

GREATER FLEXIBILITY

Once your spine has become more supple, you can make this a continuous movement. Hollow your spine as you breathe in. Then, without holding the position, immediately arch your back while breathing out. Repeat ten times, following the rhythm of your breathing. When you have finished, lower yourself into the *Child* pose *(see page 62)* and relax, breathing normally, for several minutes.

The Bridge

Setu Bandhasana, the Bridge, is a powerful backward stretch that strengthens the neck and spine and helps to tighten the muscles of the abdomen. Although it may look formidable, it is actually quite a simple posture. There are two methods of coming into this posture. The technique for beginners is shown here, while intermediate students may start from a full Shoulder Stand (*see page 150*).

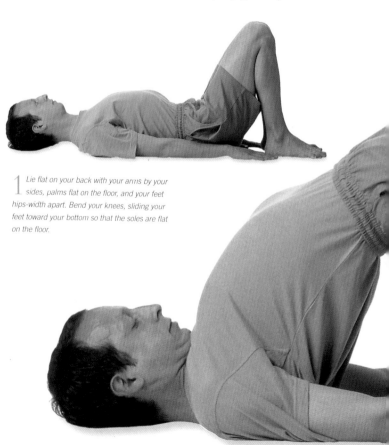

1 Lie flat on your back with your arms by your sides, palms flat on the floor, and your feet hips-width apart. Bend your knees, sliding your feet toward your bottom so that the soles are flat on the floor.

SPINAL MOBILITY

Supporting your back with your hands makes it easier if you are little stiff and your back is not very mobile. Start from the position described in Step 1. As you breathe in, bend your elbows and slide your palms beneath the small of your back. Ideally, do this with your fingers pointing toward your spine, but if you find another position more comfortable, use that to begin with. While breathing out, raise your hips, chest, and thighs as high as possible, supporting the small of your back with your hands. Keep your shoulders, neck, and head flat on the ground and don't let your knees spread apart. Breathing normally, hold for a count of ten, then gently lower your chest and hips to the floor, sliding your hands back to your sides. When you can hold the *Bridge* in this position for at least a count of 30, try it without supporting your back with your hands.

2 While breathing in, press down with your arms and feet and lift your hips, chest, and thighs as high as possible, without straining. Keep your head, neck, and shoulders flat on the ground and do not come up on to your toes. Breathing normally, hold for a count of ten, gradually building up to a count of 30. Breathing out, lower your chest and hips to the floor, then rest with your knees bent.

WATCHPOINT

Not suitable for people with neck, throat, or upper back conditions. Also, stop immediately if you experience any pain.

The King Pigeon

The several *Kapotasanas,* or Pigeon postures, are all backward bends
that stretch the entire body, improve the spine's flexibility, and
stimulate circulation. In this simplified version, the extended leg
stays straight behind the body and the bent leg and foot are kept in
front. From a side view, the chest looks puffed out like a pigeon.

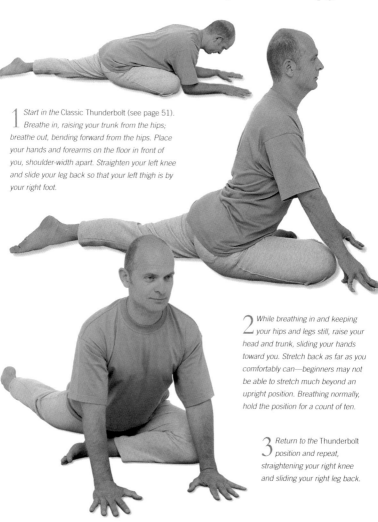

1 *Start in the* Classic Thunderbolt *(see page 51).
Breathe in, raising your trunk from the hips;
breathe out, bending forward from the hips. Place
your hands and forearms on the floor in front of
you, shoulder-width apart. Straighten your left knee
and slide your leg back so that your left thigh is by
your right foot.*

2 *While breathing in and keeping
your hips and legs still, raise your
head and trunk, sliding your hands
toward you. Stretch back as far as you
comfortably can—beginners may not
be able to stretch much beyond an
upright position. Breathing normally,
hold the position for a count of ten.*

3 *Return to the* Thunderbolt
*position and repeat,
straightening your right knee
and sliding your right leg back.*

The Half Locust

As well as increasing the flexibility of the upper back, *Ardha-Salabhasana* strengthens the abdominal muscles and helps regulate the digestive system. Beneficial to people who suffer from varicose veins, it also expands the chest, making it helpful for those with respiratory problems.

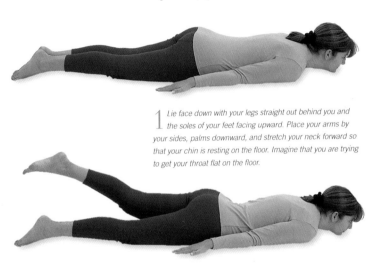

1 *Lie face down with your legs straight out behind you and the soles of your feet facing upward. Place your arms by your sides, palms downward, and stretch your neck forward so that your chin is resting on the floor. Imagine that you are trying to get your throat flat on the floor.*

2 *As you breathe in, gently raise your left leg, keeping it completely straight. Do not twist your hips or lift your chin off the floor. You may not be able to lift your leg very high, but do not force or jerk it. Holding your breath, keep this position for a count of five, if possible. Then, as you breathe out, gently lower your leg. Repeat with your right leg. Then repeat the whole exercise twice more.*

THE LOCUST

Once you are confident with the *Half Locust,* try the full *Locust.* Start as in Step 1, but clench your fists. Take three deep breaths and, on the final one, raise both legs together as high as possible, keeping your elbows straight and your shoulders and chin on the floor. Do not twist your hips. Breathing normally, hold the position for a count of five, gradually building up to a count of 30. As you breathe out, lower your legs and unclench your fists. Rest and repeat.

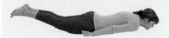

WATCHPOINT
Not suitable for pregnant women.

The Cobra

Bhujangasana mimics the action of the hooded cobra about to strike. It stimulates the circulation, increases the flexibility of the spine, and tones the back muscles. The gentle pressure on the abdominal organs can relieve menstrual problems. It is a powerful backward bend, so should always be countered by a forward bend.

ADVANCED COBRA

Start as in Step 1, but place the hands, palms downward and fingers pointing forward, directly beneath your shoulders. Tuck in your elbows. Gently roll your head upward—as your forehead moves up, your nose and then your chin should touch the floor. Keep pushing your chin forward as you roll your body up and back as far as it will go. Your elbows should remain slightly bent and you should not use your arms to push your body up. Keep your knees straight and your legs and hips flat on the floor. Breathing normally, hold the position for a count of ten, slowly building up to 60. Then gradually roll back down in reverse order.

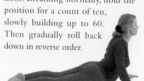

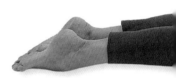

1 Lie face down with your legs together and straight behind you. Keep your legs relaxed, your toes pointing slightly inward, and your heels out to the sides. Place your arms, palms upward, by your sides and rest your forehead on the floor.

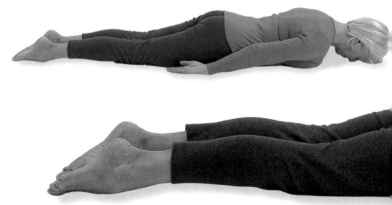

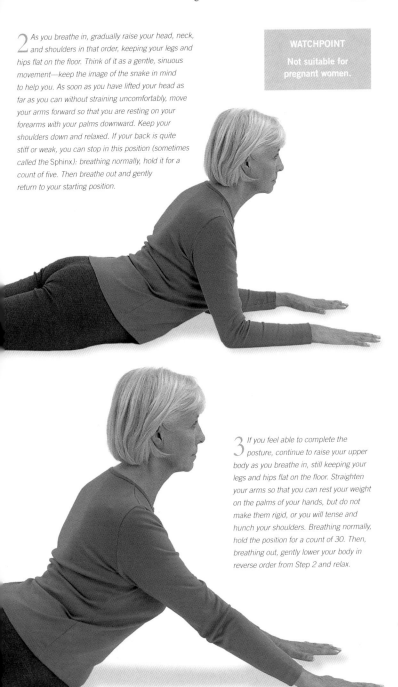

2 As you breathe in, gradually raise your head, neck, and shoulders in that order, keeping your legs and hips flat on the floor. Think of it as a gentle, sinuous movement—keep the image of the snake in mind to help you. As soon as you have lifted your head as far as you can without straining uncomfortably, move your arms forward so that you are resting on your forearms with your palms downward. Keep your shoulders down and relaxed. If your back is quite stiff or weak, you can stop in this position (sometimes called the Sphinx): breathing normally, hold it for a count of five. Then breathe out and gently return to your starting position.

WATCHPOINT
Not suitable for
pregnant women.

3 If you feel able to complete the posture, continue to raise your upper body as you breathe in, still keeping your legs and hips flat on the floor. Straighten your arms so that you can rest your weight on the palms of your hands, but do not make them rigid, or you will tense and hunch your shoulders. Breathing normally, hold the position for a count of 30. Then, breathing out, gently lower your body in reverse order from Step 2 and relax.

The Dog

A full-body stretch, this strengthens the muscles of the
neck, back, hips, abdomen, and legs and stimulates circulation.
It is a very relaxing pose and increases your vitality. Use
it to counter backward bends.

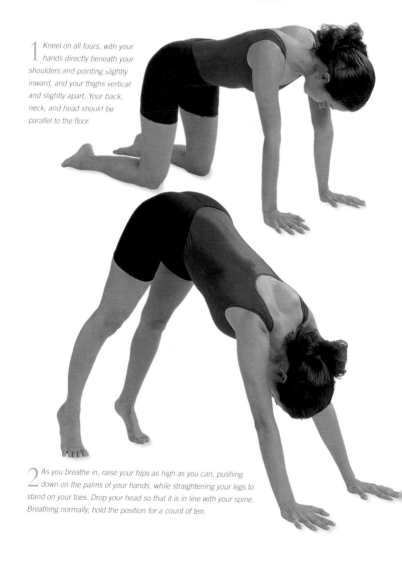

1 Kneel on all fours, with your
hands directly beneath your
shoulders and pointing slightly
inward, and your thighs vertical
and slightly apart. Your back,
neck, and head should be
parallel to the floor.

2 As you breathe in, raise your hips as high as you can, pushing
down on the palms of your hands, while straightening your legs to
stand on your toes. Drop your head so that it is in line with your spine.
Breathing normally, hold the position for a count of ten.

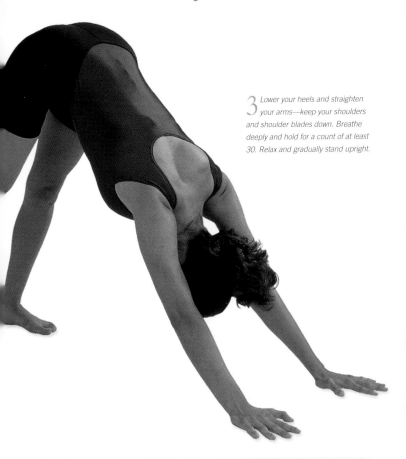

3 Lower your heels and straighten your arms—keep your shoulders and shoulder blades down. Breathe deeply and hold for a count of at least 30. Relax and gradually stand upright.

FLEXING THE ANKLES AND KNEES

You can add an extra step to help loosen up the joints of the lower leg and further strengthen the calf muscles.

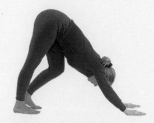

Before relaxing at the end of Step 3, press your right heel firmly into the floor, then raise your left heel and bend your left knee.

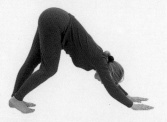

Press your left heel firmly into the floor, then raise your right heel and bend your right knee. Repeat these steps several times, then relax.

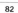

The Cow Pose

This pose stretches the legs, increases the flexibility of the hips, and improves balance. When you are learning the pose, you may find it helpful to sit with your back against a wall.

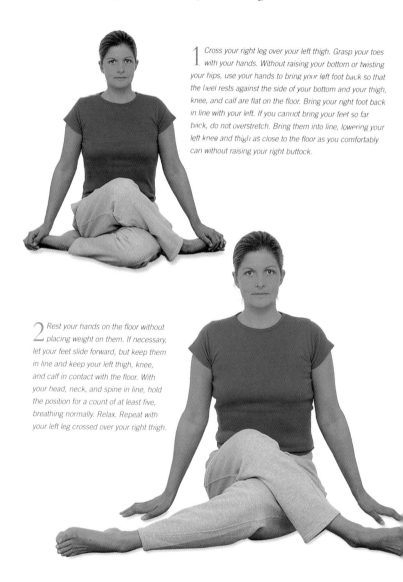

1 Cross your right leg over your left thigh. Grasp your toes with your hands. Without raising your bottom or twisting your hips, use your hands to bring your left foot back so that the heel rests against the side of your bottom and your thigh, knee, and calf are flat on the floor. Bring your right foot back in line with your left. If you cannot bring your feet so far back, do not overstretch. Bring them into line, lowering your left knee and thigh as close to the floor as you comfortably can without raising your right buttock.

2 Rest your hands on the floor without placing weight on them. If necessary, let your feet slide forward, but keep them in line and keep your left thigh, knee, and calf in contact with the floor. With your head, neck, and spine in line, hold the position for a count of at least five, breathing normally. Relax. Repeat with your left leg crossed over your right thigh.

The Head of a Cow

Also known as the Face of a Cow, this posture is said to resemble a cow's head when viewed from behind. It improves posture, tones the muscles of the shoulders and upper back, strengthens the triceps muscles in the upper arms, and loosens the shoulder joints. You can do this in the Cow (*see opposite*), the Classic Thunderbolt (*see page 51*), or even seated on a chair.

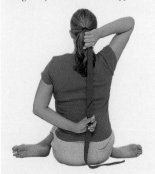

1 *Start in your chosen position. Bend your right arm, raising your elbow, then stretch your hand over your right shoulder and down the middle of your back as far as possible. Keeping your head, neck, and spine in line, bend your left arm and bring your left hand up the middle of your back until the fingers of both hands meet.*

2 *Curl the fingers of your left and right hands together, hooking them firmly—keep the palm of your right hand toward your back and the palm of your left hand facing outward. Breathing normally, hold for a count of at least six, then relax. Repeat with your arms in reverse positions.*

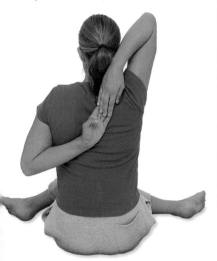

STIFF SHOULDERS

If your shoulder joints are not sufficiently flexible to enable you to interlock your hands, grip a belt or handkerchief, gradually decreasing its length as you become more supple.

The Cobbler

Baddha Konasana is known both as the Cobbler, because
of the way Indian cobblers traditionally sit, and the Butterfly,
because of the shape your legs form. It is also called *Bhadrasana,*
the Auspicious Posture. It stretches the inner thighs and hips,
relieving tension in the lower back. It increases flexibility in the
ankles, knees, and hips; tones the urinary and reproductive systems;
and is a preparatory step toward learning the more advanced Half
Lotus and Lotus poses (*see pages 86–87*).

1 *Sit on the floor with your legs
straight in front of you. Stretch
your trunk up from your hips, rather
than slumping on the base of your
spine. Bend your knees and bring
the soles of your feet together.*

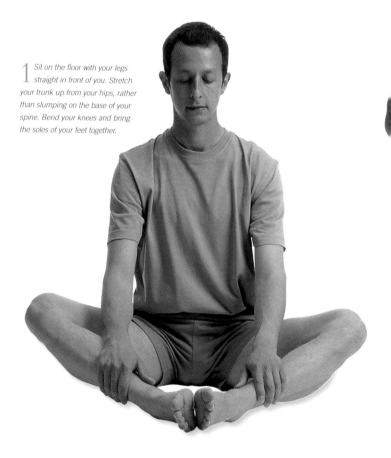

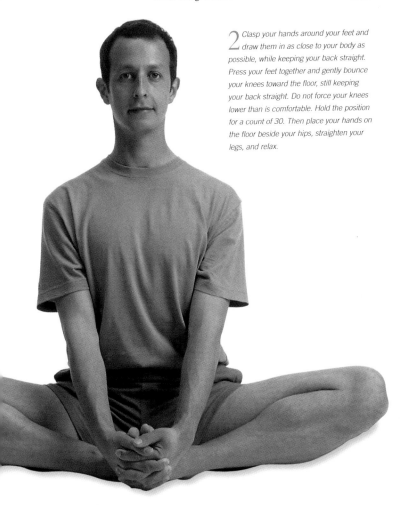

2 Clasp your hands around your feet and draw them in as close to your body as possible, while keeping your back straight. Press your feet together and gently bounce your knees toward the floor, still keeping your back straight. Do not force your knees lower than is comfortable. Hold the position for a count of 30. Then place your hands on the floor beside your hips, straighten your legs, and relax.

EASING THE STRETCH

Westerners unused to sitting on the floor tend to have quite stiff hips, although anyone trained as a dancer will find this pose fairly easy. If your knees don't seem to bounce anywhere near the floor, try sitting on a foam block or even two, or on a folded rug. This will make it easier for you to stretch your trunk upward from the lower back and to get your knees lower down. Even so, when you're doing this be careful not to strain your groin. As your hips become more flexible, you can dispense with the foam blocks or rug.

The Half Lotus

This pose, *Ardha-Padmasana,* is an intermediary stage between the Cobbler (*see pages 84–85*) and the Lotus, the classic pose for meditation. It increases flexibility in the ankles, knees, and hips, but they should already be fairly mobile before you try it. If you can sit cross-legged for at least ten minutes, without feeling any strain or discomfort, then you can probably try the Half Lotus.

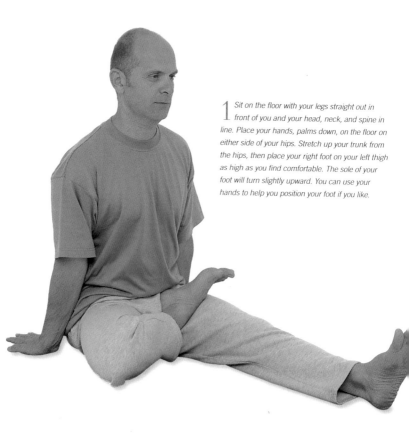

1 *Sit on the floor with your legs straight out in front of you and your head, neck, and spine in line. Place your hands, palms down, on the floor on either side of your hips. Stretch up your trunk from the hips, then place your right foot on your left thigh as high as you find comfortable. The sole of your foot will turn slightly upward. You can use your hands to help you position your foot if you like.*

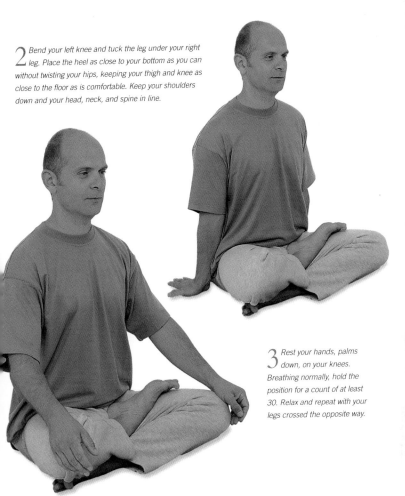

2 Bend your left knee and tuck the leg under your right leg. Place the heel as close to your bottom as you can without twisting your hips, keeping your thigh and knee as close to the floor as is comfortable. Keep your shoulders down and your head, neck, and spine in line.

3 Rest your hands, palms down, on your knees. Breathing normally, hold the position for a count of at least 30. Relax and repeat with your legs crossed the opposite way.

THE LOTUS

Some people progress easily from half to full *Lotus*, while others find it quite difficult. As it is easy to cause strain and to develop bad habits, such as a rounded or twisted back or hunched shoulders, it is best learned with a teacher. It is not recommended for beginners. Starting from the *Easy* position (*see page 50*), the left foot is placed on the right thigh as high as feels comfortable—the sole will automatically turn so that it faces upward. The left knee rests on the floor. Then the right foot is brought up on to the left thigh with the right knee resting on the floor. The head, neck, and spine remain straight and erect. For meditation, the hands may be placed in *Chin Mudra* (*see page 50*) or rested in the lap, one inside the other with the palms facing upward. *Lotus* can, of course, also be done the other way round, positioning the right foot first.

The Hero

Virasana, the Hero pose, is a perfect example of the difficulties modern authorities have in interpreting the classic texts, which, in any case, do not always agree with each other. There are at least six versions of this basic pose. This one is a simple, resting posture that soothes the mind and acts as an antidote to stress. In fact, some authorities call it the Resting Hero.

1 *Kneel down with your knees almost touching, your feet hips-width apart, and your arms by your sides. Keep your back, neck, and head in line. If your knees are a bit creaky, kneel on a mat or blanket.*

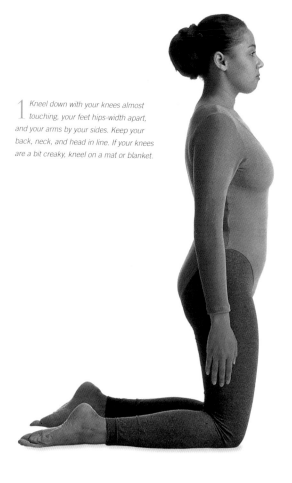

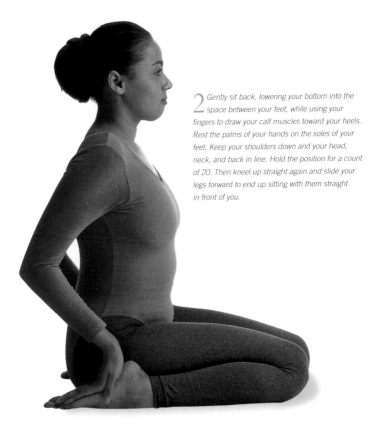

2 Gently sit back, lowering your bottom into the space between your feet, while using your fingers to draw your calf muscles toward your heels. Rest the palms of your hands on the soles of your feet. Keep your shoulders down and your head, neck, and back in line. Hold the position for a count of 20. Then kneel up straight again and slide your legs forward to end up sitting with them straight in front of you.

THE SUPINE HERO

Supta Virasana, Supine Hero, is an extreme stretch involving the muscles of the thighs, knees, and ankles. It improves spinal flexibility, opens up the chest, and stimulates the circulation. It is not recommended for beginners, but those who are already fairly supple find it intensely therapeutic. If it helps, place a pillow under the small of your back or under the back of your knees.

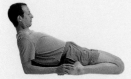

1 Sit in the Hero pose. Then, as you breathe out, bend back from your hips until your trunk rests on your elbows. Keep your hands on the soles of your feet and your back straight.

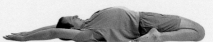

2 Lower your back until your head is resting on the floor. Stretch your arms to the side and then stretch them behind your head, palms facing upward. Breathe deeply and hold the position for at least a count of 20. With practice, you will able to hold the position for ten minutes or more. Then return to the Hero pose and relax.

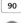

The Gate

This pose is named after the Sanskrit word *parigha*, which means the bar used for locking a gate. *Parighasana* is sometimes translated as the Locked Gate pose. It is quite a powerful sideways stretch that strengthens the muscles of the waist and helps trim superfluous fat.

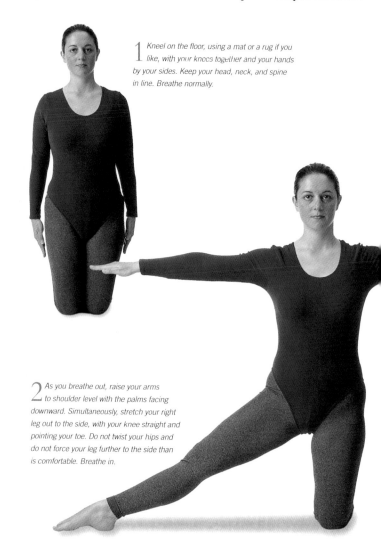

1 Kneel on the floor, using a mat or a rug if you like, with your knees together and your hands by your sides. Keep your head, neck, and spine in line. Breathe normally.

2 As you breathe out, raise your arms to shoulder level with the palms facing downward. Simultaneously, stretch your right leg out to the side, with your knee straight and pointing your toe. Do not twist your hips and do not force your leg further to the side than is comfortable. Breathe in.

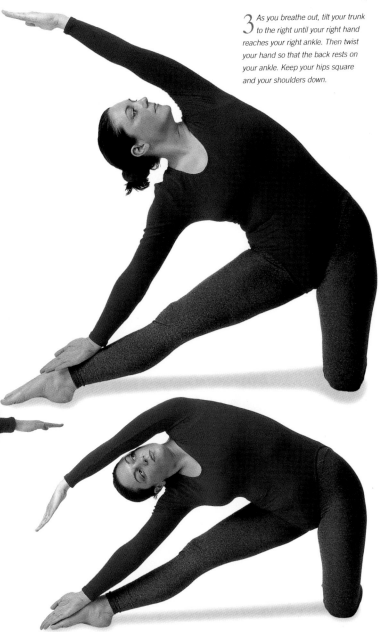

3 *As you breathe out, tilt your trunk to the right until your right hand reaches your right ankle. Then twist your hand so that the back rests on your ankle. Keep your hips square and your shoulders down.*

4 *Facing forward, gently swing your left arm further over until your upper arm rests on your left ear. Breathing normally, hold the position for a count of ten, gradually building up to a count of 20. Return to the kneeling position of Step 1 and repeat on the left.*

Supine Twist

This is a gentle spinal stretch and twist that helps tone the muscles of the lower back. Roll your knees only as far as is comfortable without forcing them—stop immediately if you feel any pain. Until your spine becomes flexible, you will probably find that you can roll them further on one side than the other.

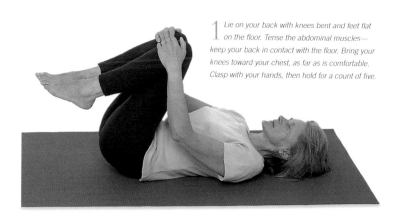

1 Lie on your back with knees bent and feet flat on the floor. Tense the abdominal muscles— keep your back in contact with the floor. Bring your knees toward your chest, as far as is comfortable. Clasp with your hands, then hold for a count of five.

2 Return to the starting position. Stretch out your arms to the sides in line with your shoulders. As you breathe in, gently and slowly roll your knees to the left, while turning your head to the right. Breathing normally, hold for a count of five. Slowly roll your knees back to the starting position. Repeat, rolling to the right.

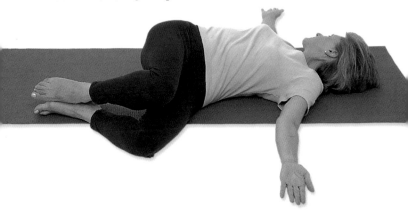

Revolving Abdomen

Jathara Parivartanasana is sometimes less elegantly, but just as accurately, translated as the Belly-Turning posture. It can be practiced in the beginner's version shown here, or a more advanced one with straight legs. It strengthens the back and tones the abdominal muscles, helping to remove superfluous fat from the waistline. It also benefits a number of internal organs, including the liver and the intestines.

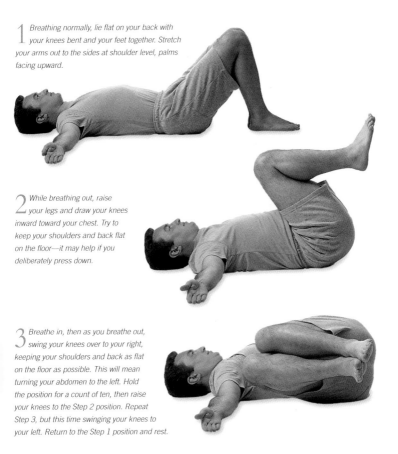

1 Breathing normally, lie flat on your back with your knees bent and your feet together. Stretch your arms out to the sides at shoulder level, palms facing upward.

2 While breathing out, raise your legs and draw your knees inward toward your chest. Try to keep your shoulders and back flat on the floor—it may help if you deliberately press down.

3 Breathe in, then as you breathe out, swing your knees over to your right, keeping your shoulders and back as flat on the floor as possible. This will mean turning your abdomen to the left. Hold the position for a count of ten, then raise your knees to the Step 2 position. Repeat Step 3, but this time swinging your knees to your left. Return to the Step 1 position and rest.

Simple Spinal Twist

This is an exhilarating way to tone the muscles of the back, loosen the shoulders, and add elasticity to the spine. It helps to prevent back problems, such as lumbago, from developing and can alleviate back pain. However, if doing this twist makes your back hurt, you should stop immediately.

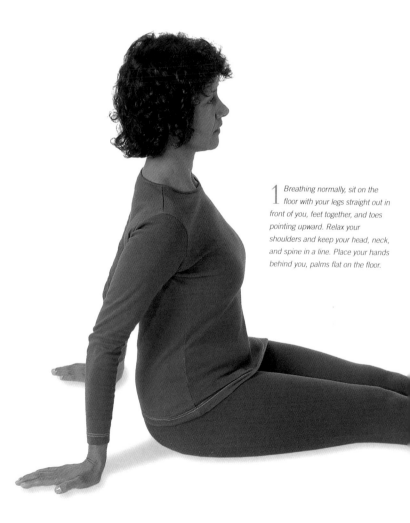

1 Breathing normally, sit on the floor with your legs straight out in front of you, feet together, and toes pointing upward. Relax your shoulders and keep your head, neck, and spine in a line. Place your hands behind you, palms flat on the floor.

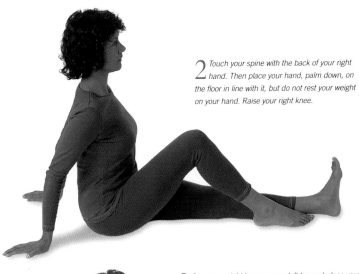

2 *Touch your spine with the back of your right hand. Then place your hand, palm down, on the floor in line with it, but do not rest your weight on your hand. Raise your right knee.*

3 *Cross your right leg over your left leg and place your right foot flat on the floor beside your left knee. Place your left hand on your left shin with your elbow pressing against the outside of your right knee. As you breathe out, turn your shoulders as far as you can to the right, keeping your back straight and your shoulders down, and without putting your weight on your right hand.*
Breathing normally, hold the position for a count of 60, then return to the position in Step 1. Repeat, crossing your left leg over your right.

HALF AND FULL SPINAL TWISTS

When you feel confident about your spine's flexibility, you can try a half twist. This is very similar to the *Simple Spinal Twist*, but before you cross your right leg over your left leg in Step 2, bend your left knee, tucking your heel in tight against your bottom. Extend your arm in Step 3 so that you can press your elbow against your right knee. In the full *Spinal Twist*, the left knee is bent and the left foot placed high up on the right thigh in Step 2. It is an advanced pose, requiring flexible hips as well as a flexible spine.

The Simple Sage

There are several *Marichyasanas,* or Sage poses. This one is suitable for beginners, but if your spine is not yet very flexible or your shoulders are quite stiff, you may find the twist and powerful stretch of the entire trunk uncomfortable or painful. If so, stop and concentrate on a less strenuous pose, such as the Simple Spinal Twist (*see pages 94–95*), until your back muscles and spine are more elastic. This position will strengthen the back and abdominal muscles and increase the blood supply to the kidneys.

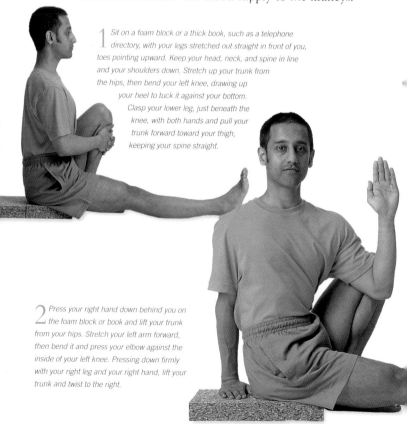

1 *Sit on a foam block or a thick book, such as a telephone directory, with your legs stretched out straight in front of you, toes pointing upward. Keep your head, neck, and spine in line and your shoulders down. Stretch up your trunk from the hips, then bend your left knee, drawing up your heel to tuck it against your bottom. Clasp your lower leg, just beneath the knee, with both hands and pull your trunk forward toward your thigh, keeping your spine straight.*

2 *Press your right hand down behind you on the foam block or book and lift your trunk from your hips. Stretch your left arm forward, then bend it and press your elbow against the inside of your left knee. Pressing down firmly with your right leg and your right hand, lift your trunk and twist to the right.*

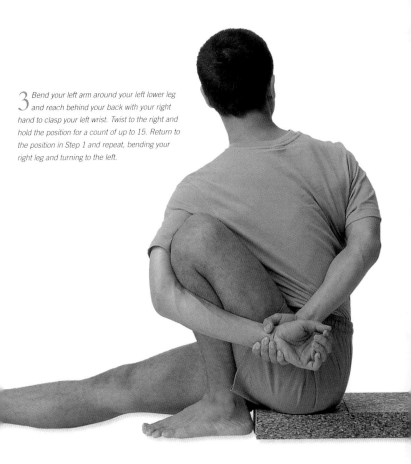

3 Bend your left arm around your left lower leg and reach behind your back with your right hand to clasp your left wrist. Twist to the right and hold the position for a count of up to 15. Return to the position in Step 1 and repeat, bending your right leg and turning to the left.

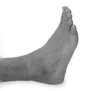

A HEALTHY SPINE

A healthy spine is crucial to physical and mental well-being. We tend to think of the spine as simply a series of bones, but the spinal cord contains a vital fluid that provides the brain and nerves with nutrients and oxygen and so affects every cell in the body. Spinal twists, such as the *Simple Sage*, help to counteract tension in the back and any tendency to slump— something most of us do when we're tired or fed up. They also increase the healthy flow of the cerebrospinal fluid. After practicing spinal twists, you will feel re-energized and alert and will no longer feel fed up or grumpy. Always include one twist—to both the left and right—in your daily yoga practice.

The Reverse Sage

When you feel confident with the Simple Sage (*see pages 96–97*), you can try this pose. Also, beginners who want to achieve greater flexibility of the spine can practice the first two steps of both Sage poses without risking strain. The health benefits of this pose are the same as those for the Simple Sage.

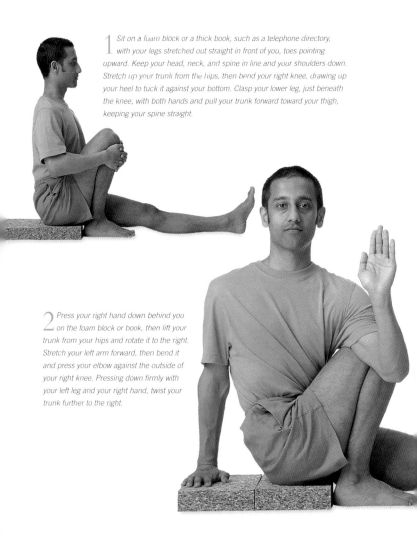

1 Sit on a foam block or a thick book, such as a telephone directory, with your legs stretched out straight in front of you, toes pointing upward. Keep your head, neck, and spine in line and your shoulders down. Stretch up your trunk from the hips, then bend your right knee, drawing up your heel to tuck it against your bottom. Clasp your lower leg, just beneath the knee, with both hands and pull your trunk forward toward your thigh, keeping your spine straight.

2 Press your right hand down behind you on the foam block or book, then lift your trunk from your hips and rotate it to the right. Stretch your left arm forward, then bend it and press your elbow against the outside of your right knee. Pressing down firmly with your left leg and your right hand, twist your trunk further to the right.

THE SAGE IN HALF LOTUS

An advanced version of the *Sage*, this helps to tone the nervous system, improve concentration, and strengthen ankle joints. Sit on the floor, your legs stretched out in front of you, toes pointing upward. Bend the left knee and draw the leg toward you, tucking your heel against your bottom. Clasp your lower leg beneath the knee and pull your trunk forward toward your thigh. Place your right foot as high as is comfortable on your left thigh, then press your right hand down behind you and lift your trunk from the hips. Stretch your left arm forward, then bend it, and press the elbow against the inside of your left knee. Lift your trunk and twist to the right. Bend your left arm around your left lower leg, then reach behind your back with your right hand to clasp your left wrist.

3 Bend your left arm around your right lower leg and reach behind you to clasp your left wrist between your thumb and fingers. Hold the position for a count of 15. Then return to the position in Step 1 and repeat, bending your left leg and turning to the left.

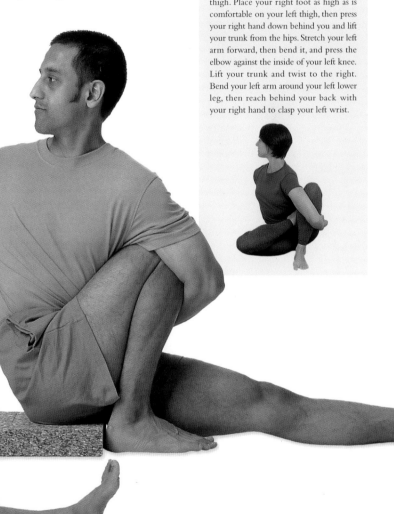

Cross-Legged Twist

Like the Simple Spinal Twist (*see pages 94–95*), this is a good way to tone the muscles of the back and neck and to keep the spine elastic. Regular practice will relieve pain in the lower back. However, if doing this twist makes your back hurt, you should stop immediately. It is also beneficial to the liver and spleen; aids the digestive system; and promotes a positive state of mind.

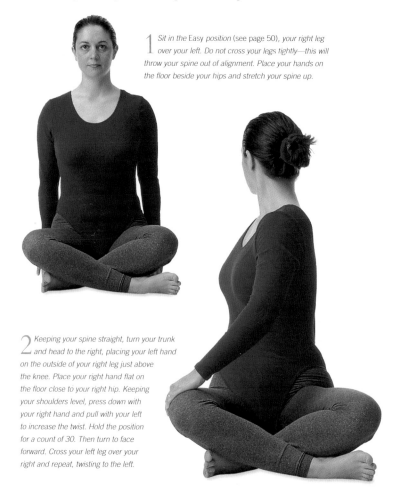

1 *Sit in the Easy position (see page 50), your right leg over your left. Do not cross your legs tightly—this will throw your spine out of alignment. Place your hands on the floor beside your hips and stretch your spine up.*

2 *Keeping your spine straight, turn your trunk and head to the right, placing your left hand on the outside of your right leg just above the knee. Place your right hand flat on the floor close to your right hip. Keeping your shoulders level, press down with your right hand and pull with your left to increase the twist. Hold the position for a count of 30. Then turn to face forward. Cross your left leg over your right and repeat, twisting to the left.*

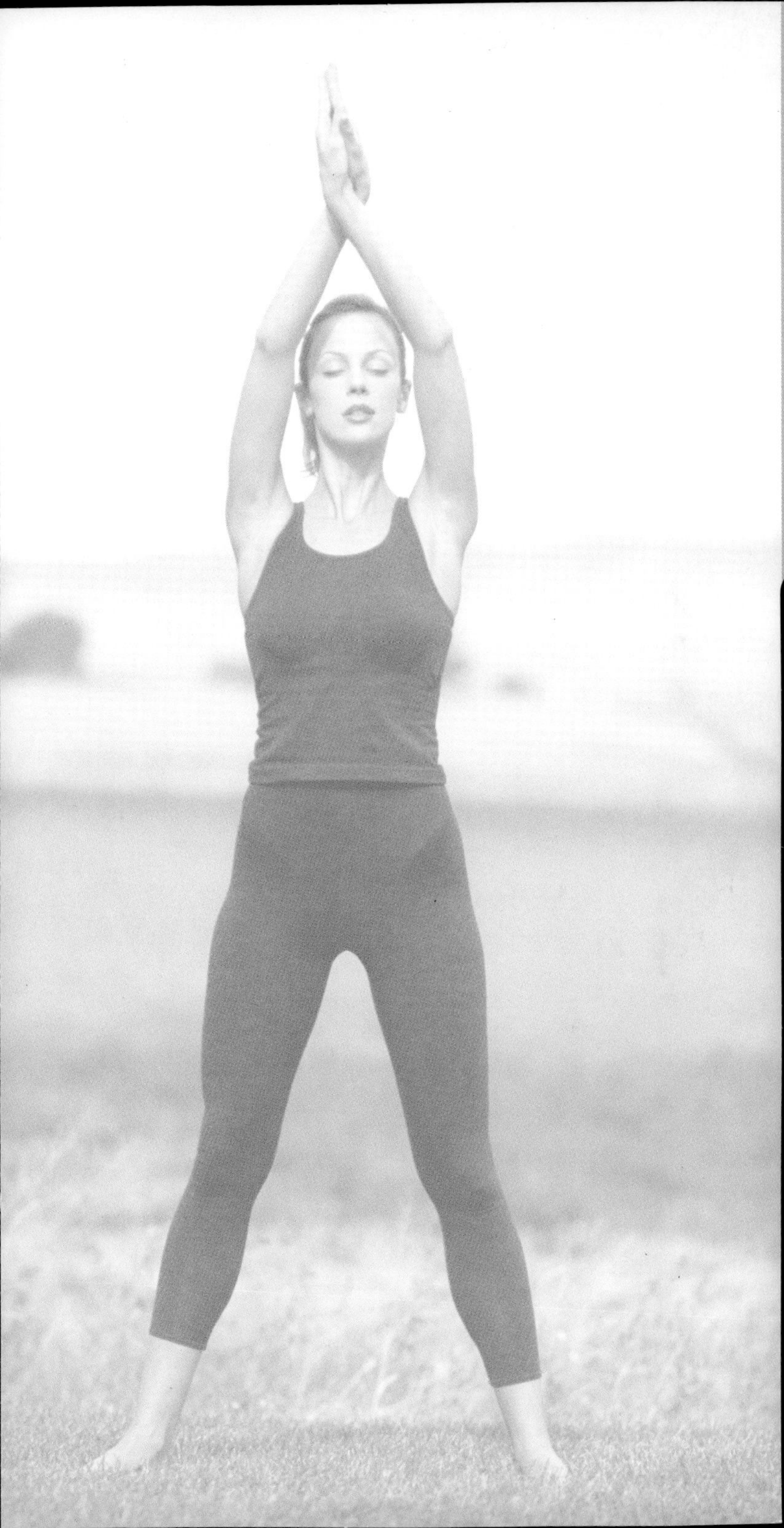

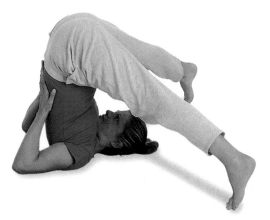

Further Poses

It is interesting to learn new poses and also fun, partly because this helps prevent complacency when practicing. With familiarity, it can be tempting to "go through the motions" in the poses rather than focus, concentrating fully on each step. Introduce new poses gradually into your practice and don't feel that you have to master every single one. Not all the poses in this chapter are intermediate or advanced. Some are suitable for beginners. As before, don't try to force your body into a posture that it is not yet capable of achieving or that causes discomfort or pain. Progressing along the yoga path at your own pace will be much more rewarding than racing to the end.

Triangle Forward Bend

This is one of many variations of the Triangle (*see pages 70–71*),
stretching the muscles and joints of the hip and legs and the sides
of the abdomen and chest. Placing the hands in the Prayer position
(*see page 58*) behind you, strengthens the muscles of the chest,
shoulders, and arms. In a similar and slightly more demanding
variation, the hands are clasped behind the back and then raised
as high as possible without bending the elbows in the final step.

1 Start in the Upright
Steadiness (see page 51).
Place your hands behind you
with your fingertips touching
and pointing downward.

2 Keeping your fingertips together, turn
your hands inward through 180°, so
that your fingers point upward. Press your
elbows back and stretch them downward,
lifting your hands and forearms to press
your hands flat together.

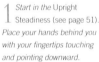

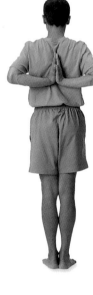

3 Breathing in, jump your feet apart sideways
to a distance of 3½–4 feet/1–1.2 meters,
keeping your hands in the Prayer position.

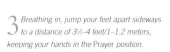

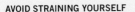

AVOID STRAINING YOURSELF

This is an intensive stretch. If you cannot bend forward sufficiently to touch your leg, bend only as far as is comfortable. Do not bend your knees or lift your back heel instead. With plenty of regular practice, you will eventually be able to touch your lower leg with your face, keeping your head, neck, and spine in line.

4 Breathing normally, turn your left foot inward and your right foot and leg out to the right, so that your heels are at right angles to each other and your right heel is aligned with your left instep. Press your left heel down and stretch both legs up from the feet without "locking" your knees. Turn your hips and trunk to the right. Stretch your trunk up from the hips, keeping your head, neck, and spine in line. Breathe in deeply.

5 While breathing out, bend forward from your hips until your face touches your lower leg. Keep your left foot flat on the floor and your left leg straight. Hold the position for at least a count of ten, breathing normally. While breathing in, raise your trunk and turn your trunk, hips, and feet to face forward, with your hands still in the Prayer position. Turn your feet to the left and repeat Steps 4 and 5.

The Palm Tree

This is one of a number of *Palmyrasanas* that were all designed to stretch the muscles in the sides of the trunk and make the spine more flexible. This particular version boosts circulation to the internal organs and helps open up the chest and lungs. It is also a useful posture to include in your warming-up routine.

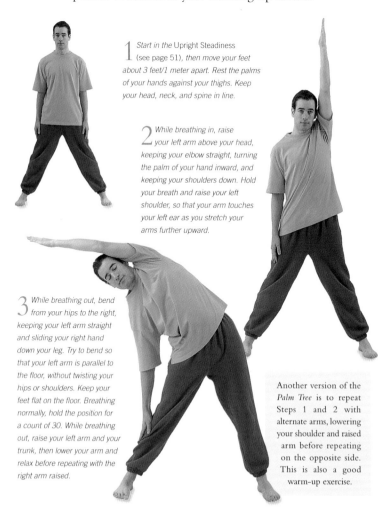

1 *Start in the* Upright Steadiness *(see page 51), then move your feet about 3 feet/1 meter apart. Rest the palms of your hands against your thighs. Keep your head, neck, and spine in line.*

2 *While breathing in, raise your left arm above your head, keeping your elbow straight, turning the palm of your hand inward, and keeping your shoulders down. Hold your breath and raise your left shoulder, so that your arm touches your left ear as you stretch your arms further upward.*

3 *While breathing out, bend from your hips to the right, keeping your left arm straight and sliding your right hand down your leg. Try to bend so that your left arm is parallel to the floor, without twisting your hips or shoulders. Keep your feet flat on the floor. Breathing normally, hold the position for a count of 30. While breathing out, raise your left arm and your trunk, then lower your arm and relax before repeating with the right arm raised.*

Another version of the *Palm Tree* is to repeat Steps 1 and 2 with alternate arms, lowering your shoulder and raised arm before repeating on the opposite side. This is also a good warm-up exercise.

Stretched Side Angle

Utthita Parvsvakonasna was devised by the Indian teacher B. K. S. Iyengar—*utthita* means stretched; *parsva*, side; and *kona*, angle. It tones and strengthens the leg muscles; strengthens the ankle and knee joints; expands the chest; and stretches the muscles of the arms, shoulders, and back. It encourages the blood supply to the spinal nerves and abdominal organs and may ease constipation. It also gets rid of superfluous fat from the hips and waist.

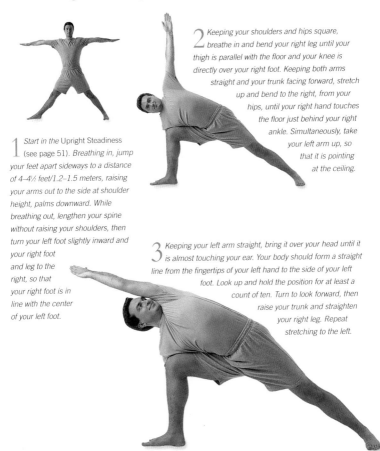

1 *Start in the* Upright Steadiness *(see page 51). Breathing in, jump your feet apart sideways to a distance of 4–4½ feet/1.2–1.5 meters, raising your arms out to the side at shoulder height, palms downward. While breathing out, lengthen your spine without raising your shoulders, then turn your left foot slightly inward and your right foot and leg to the right, so that your right foot is in line with the center of your left foot.*

2 *Keeping your shoulders and hips square, breathe in and bend your right leg until your thigh is parallel with the floor and your knee is directly over your right foot. Keeping both arms straight and your trunk facing forward, stretch up and bend to the right, from your hips, until your right hand touches the floor just behind your right ankle. Simultaneously, take your left arm up, so that it is pointing at the ceiling.*

3 *Keeping your left arm straight, bring it over your head until it is almost touching your ear. Your body should form a straight line from the fingertips of your left hand to the side of your left foot. Look up and hold the position for at least a count of ten. Turn to look forward, then raise your trunk and straighten your right leg. Repeat stretching to the left.*

Simple Forward Bend

This is a very relaxing position that loosens tension in the back and shoulders and gently stretches the muscles and tendons in the thighs. It is a good counter to backward bends and can be done at any time when the back and shoulders feel tight, such as after a long morning at a computer keyboard. You will need a chair or something similar that reaches to about hip height.

1 Stand about 3 feet/1 meter away from the chair back with your feet about 12 inches/30 cm apart. Make sure your weight is evenly balanced. Stretch up your legs from the ankles and, as you breathe in, raise your arms above your head, keeping your shoulders down.

2 As you breathe out, bend forward from your hips and place your hands, shoulder-width apart, on the chair back. Move your hips back in line with your feet, and lower your head so that your head, neck, and spine are in line. Do not hang on to the back of the chair or let your spine sag, and keep your legs straight and pressing back. Breathe in as you stretch your trunk forward. Then, breathing normally, hold the position for a count of 20. Raise your arms and trunk and stand briefly in the Upright Steadiness (see page 51).

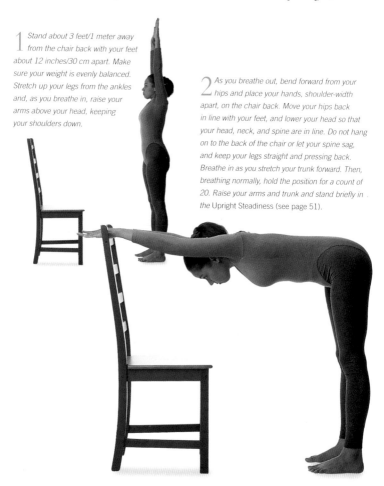

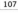

Standing Forward Bend

Uttanasana is a good way to relax between more strenuous postures and is a counter to backward bends. It stretches the spine and increases flexibility, strengthening the muscles and tendons of the legs. As it increases the flow of blood and oxygen to the brain, it helps relieve tension and invigorate the body.

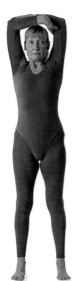

1 *Breathing normally, stand with your feet about hips-width apart and your weight evenly balanced. Stretch up from your feet and stretch up your trunk from your hips. Raise your arms above your head, keeping your shoulders down, then bend your elbows and grasp your upper arms just above the elbows.*

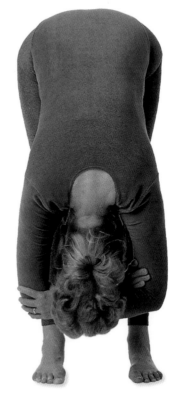

WATCHPOINT
Not recommended for sufferers with back problems or a slipped disk.

2 *Lift your elbows and, as you breathe out, bend forward from your hips. Keeping your legs stretched, lower your elbows toward the floor, letting your body relax downward and your head hang. Breathing normally, hold the position for a count of ten. Then, while breathing in, lift your head and elbows and raise your spine from your hips, sliding your hands up your legs.*

The Crescent Moon

This strong backward bend strengthens and tones the muscles of the hips, thighs, and abdomen and increases the flexibility of the spine. It also helps develop your sense of balance. The steps should flow together in a single, graceful sequence like a dance. Once you have achieved this, you will find it a very calming posture.

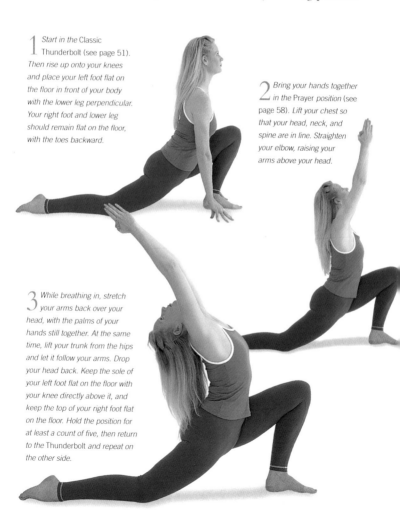

1 *Start in the* Classic Thunderbolt *(see page 51). Then rise up onto your knees and place your left foot flat on the floor in front of your body with the lower leg perpendicular. Your right foot and lower leg should remain flat on the floor, with the toes backward.*

2 *Bring your hands together in the* Prayer *position (see page 58). Lift your chest so that your head, neck, and spine are in line. Straighten your elbow, raising your arms above your head.*

3 *While breathing in, stretch your arms back over your head, with the palms of your hands still together. At the same time, lift your trunk from the hips and let it follow your arms. Drop your head back. Keep the sole of your left foot flat on the floor with your knee directly above it, and keep the top of your right foot flat on the floor. Hold the position for at least a count of five, then return to the* Thunderbolt *and repeat on the other side.*

The Powerful Pose

Utkatasana strengthens the ankles, calves, knees, and thighs and tones the muscles. It can help relieve tension and stiffness in the shoulders and also improves balance and posture generally. It is an ideal posture to practice before a skiing holiday. Beginners may find it difficult to manage this posture with their arms overhead. If so, practice with your arms held straight out, parallel to the floor.

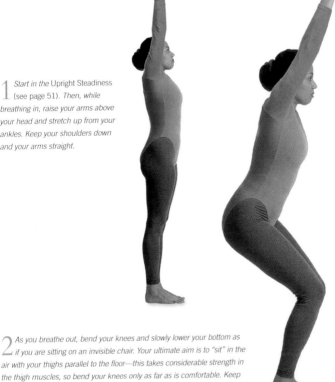

1 *Start in the* Upright Steadiness (see page 51). *Then, while breathing in, raise your arms above your head and stretch up from your ankles. Keep your shoulders down and your arms straight.*

2 *As you breathe out, bend your knees and slowly lower your bottom as if you are sitting on an invisible chair. Your ultimate aim is to "sit" in the air with your thighs parallel to the floor—this takes considerable strength in the thigh muscles, so bend your knees only as far as is comfortable. Keep your spine as straight as possible. Hold the position for a count of ten, then straighten your legs and lower your arms before repeating.*

Back Stretch

Paschimottanasana stretches the hamstrings and the muscles of the back and loosens the spine. It increases the blood supply to the spine and nervous system, as well as to the internal organs. It is thought to encourage a healthy digestive system and is reputed to increase sexual vigor and control.

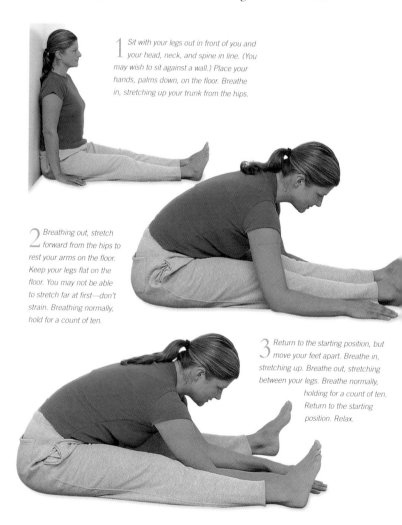

1 Sit with your legs out in front of you and your head, neck, and spine in line. (You may wish to sit against a wall.) Place your hands, palms down, on the floor. Breathe in, stretching up your trunk from the hips.

2 Breathing out, stretch forward from the hips to rest your arms on the floor. Keep your legs flat on the floor. You may not be able to stretch far at first—don't strain. Breathing normally, hold for a count of ten.

3 Return to the starting position, but move your feet apart. Breathe in, stretching up. Breathe out, stretching between your legs. Breathe normally, holding for a count of ten. Return to the starting position. Relax.

Angled Back Stretch

When you can hold the Back Stretch (*see page 110*) for a count of at least 20, try this more demanding variation. It is an intense stretch: at first, you may not be able to rest your forehead on the floor in Step 2. Position a foam block or stool in front of you and rest your forehead on that until you can complete the full pose. The health benefits are as for the Back Stretch, and the pose also opens up the chest and strengthens the neck muscles.

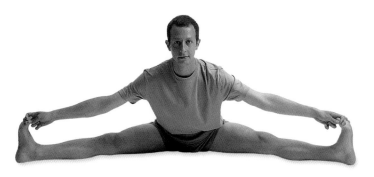

1 *Sit on the floor with your legs straight out in front of you and your head, neck, and spine in line. Place your hands, palms on the floor, on either side of your hips. Stretch up your trunk from the hips, then move your legs apart to form as wide an angle as you can without causing discomfort. Press your hands and legs into the floor and stretch up. While breathing out, bend your trunk forward from the hips and grasp the toes of your left foot with your left hand and the toes of your right foot with your right hand. Breathing normally, hold the position for a count of five. If your legs are feeling the strain, breathe in, let go of your toes, place your hands on the floor beside your hips, move your legs together—and relax. If you can comfortably hold this position for a count of 10, progress to the next step.*

2 *While breathing out, lean forward from the hips and lower your forehead as far as you can, keeping your spine straight. With practice, you will be able to rest your forehead on the floor—those who are very advanced can lower the chin and chest to the floor. Breathing normally, hold the position for a count of five. Then, while breathing in, raise your head and trunk, let go of your toes, place your hands on the floor beside your hips, move your legs together— and relax.*

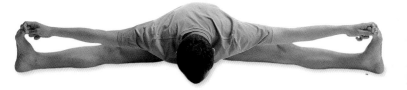

The Thunderbolt

Several valuable poses, such as the Camel (*see page 131*) and the King Pigeon (*see page 76*), begin in the Thunderbolt, so it is important to perfect it. It looks simple, but many Westerners find it difficult because they are unused to kneeling on the floor. Practice it while eating a meal Japanese-style, as it aids digestion.

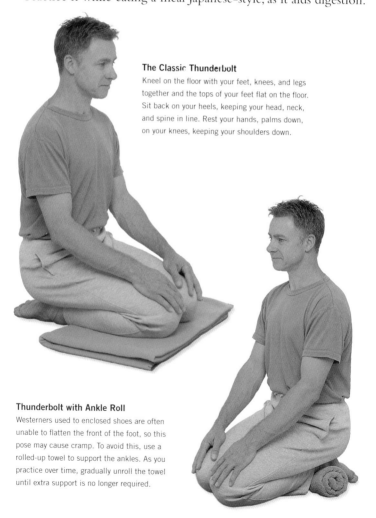

The Classic Thunderbolt
Kneel on the floor with your feet, knees, and legs together and the tops of your feet flat on the floor. Sit back on your heels, keeping your head, neck, and spine in line. Rest your hands, palms down, on your knees, keeping your shoulders down.

Thunderbolt with Ankle Roll
Westerners used to enclosed shoes are often unable to flatten the front of the foot, so this pose may cause cramp. To avoid this, use a rolled-up towel to support the ankles. As you practice over time, gradually unroll the towel until extra support is no longer required.

Thunderbolt with Tucked-Under Toes

This pose opens out the feet, and helps those with weak hamstrings or creaky knee joints. Kneel on the floor with feet, knees, and legs together. Raise your heels and tuck the toes under as if standing on tiptoe. Sit back on your heels, keeping the head, neck, and spine in line, and rest your hands on your knees.

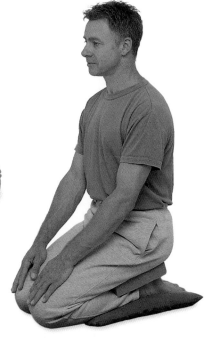

Thunderbolt with Cushions

Stiff knees or short hamstrings may make this pose hard. Use two cushions—one between the bottom and heels, one under the legs and feet. This decreases the stretch of the muscles and the leverage on the knees.

Prayer Position in Thunderbolt

Kneel in *Classic Thunderbolt*. Place your hands, palms together and fingers pointing downward, behind your back. Turn your hands in toward you and raise them until your fingers point upward. Move your hands as high up your back as possible. Strengthening the muscles of the shoulders and upper back, this counteracts a tendency to slump or hunch the shoulders.

Head–Knee Pose

Janu Sirasana is a forward bend from a sitting position. This version is sometimes called the Three-Limbed Pose, because the body is said to have three limbs when in this position—the feet, the knees, and the seat. It increases the blood supply to the spine and nervous system and to the internal organs, especially the digestive system. It strengthens the lumbar region of the back and increases spine flexibility. It is said to relieve pain and swelling in the legs and feet.

BEGINNER'S VERSION

If you find it difficult to bend your leg into the position described here, try this alternative *Head–Knee* pose. Start in the same seated position, then bend your left knee and tuck your left foot into your right thigh, so that your left lower leg is at 90° to your right thigh. Gently bounce your knee with your left hand, then press your legs down. While breathing out, lean forward from your hips, keeping your spine straight, and grasp your foot with both hands. Breathe in, pulling on your foot. Then, while breathing out, stretch your trunk along your right leg, resting your forehead on your leg. Breathing normally, hold the position. If your hips are not yet very flexible, you may find it helpful to support your bent knee with a foam block or a folded rug. If your back is still stiff, you may not be able to lower your forehead to your leg, so rest it on a thickly folded rug.

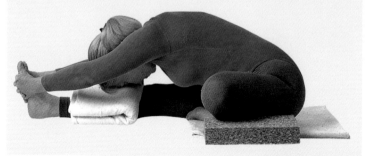

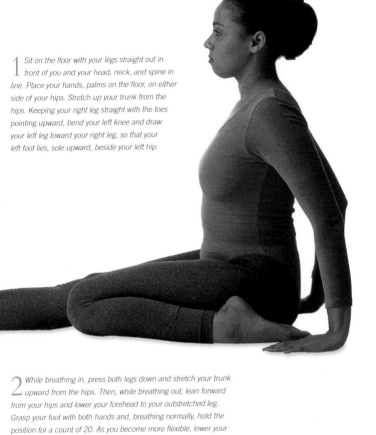

1 Sit on the floor with your legs straight out in
front of you and your head, neck, and spine in
line. Place your hands, palms on the floor, on either
side of your hips. Stretch up your trunk from the
hips. Keeping your right leg straight with the toes
pointing upward, bend your left knee and draw
your left leg toward your right leg, so that your
left foot lies, sole upward, beside your left hip.

2 While breathing in, press both legs down and stretch your trunk
upward from the hips. Then, while breathing out, lean forward
from your hips and lower your forehead to your outstretched leg.
Grasp your foot with both hands and, breathing normally, hold the
position for a count of 20. As you become more flexible, lower your
chest as well as your head onto your outstretched leg and rest your
elbows on the floor. Raise your head and release your foot, then
straighten your spine and return to the starting
position in Step 1. Repeat with
your right leg bent.

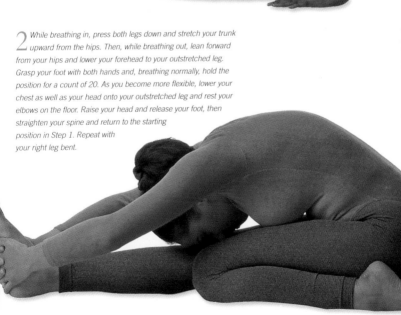

The Cross-Legged Fish

Matsyasana is a strong backward stretch of the spine and neck.
It is so called because the lungs fill with air as the chest opens out
and the center of gravity is shifted toward the center of the body,
making it a good position for floating in water. There are
a number of variations.

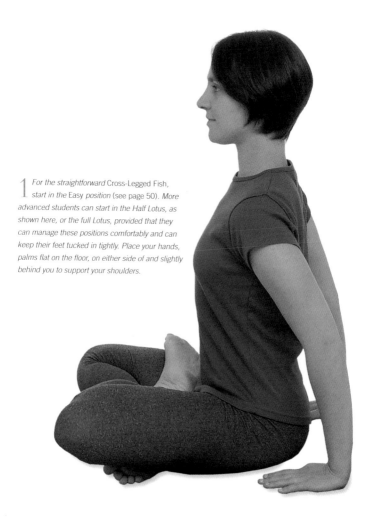

1 *For the straightforward* Cross-Legged Fish, *start in the* Easy *position (see page 50). More advanced students can start in the Half Lotus, as shown here, or the full Lotus, provided that they can manage these positions comfortably and can keep their feet tucked in tightly. Place your hands, palms flat on the floor, on either side of and slightly behind you to support your shoulders.*

2 Keeping your legs in position and your spine straight, gradually lie back onto the floor, with the head, neck, and spine in line. As you do so, bend the elbows and lower the forearms to take your weight. It may be easier to grasp your feet with your hands before lying back. If so, now rest your arms on the floor on either side of you.

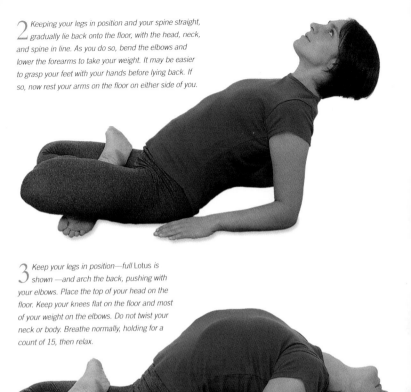

3 Keep your legs in position—full Lotus is shown —and arch the back, pushing with your elbows. Place the top of your head on the floor. Keep your knees flat on the floor and most of your weight on the elbows. Do not twist your neck or body. Breathe normally, holding for a count of 15, then relax.

THE BASIC FISH

These are advanced variations, so practice the basic pose until you can hold it for at least two minutes. Lie flat on the floor with legs and feet together and arms by your sides, palms downward. Raise your trunk to a half-sitting position, while sliding your arms back and bending your elbows. Keep the feet together and knees straight. Drop your head back until the top rests on the floor, but most of your weight is on your elbows. Your chest should be arched, but do not raise your bottom. Breathing normally, hold for a count of at least 15 seconds, then relax.

The Heron

Colorfully renamed by B. K. S. Iyengar, this traditional head-to-knee pose stretches the hamstrings; stimulates the nervous system; encourages the circulation; and benefits the digestive system. In the full pose, the forehead and chin are placed on the raised leg, while the back remains straight. Two variations are shown here.

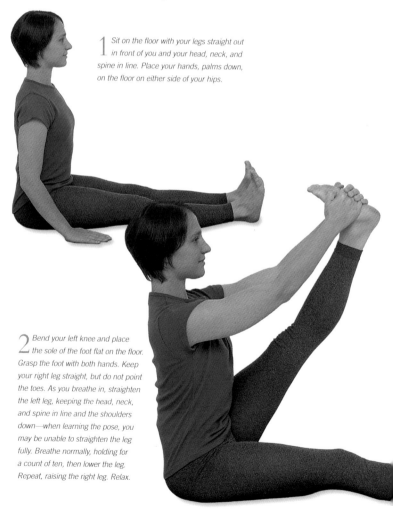

1 *Sit on the floor with your legs straight out in front of you and your head, neck, and spine in line. Place your hands, palms down, on the floor on either side of your hips.*

2 *Bend your left knee and place the sole of the foot flat on the floor. Grasp the foot with both hands. Keep your right leg straight, but do not point the toes. As you breathe in, straighten the left leg, keeping the head, neck, and spine in line and the shoulders down—when learning the pose, you may be unable to straighten the leg fully. Breathe normally, holding for a count of ten, then lower the leg. Repeat, raising the right leg. Relax.*

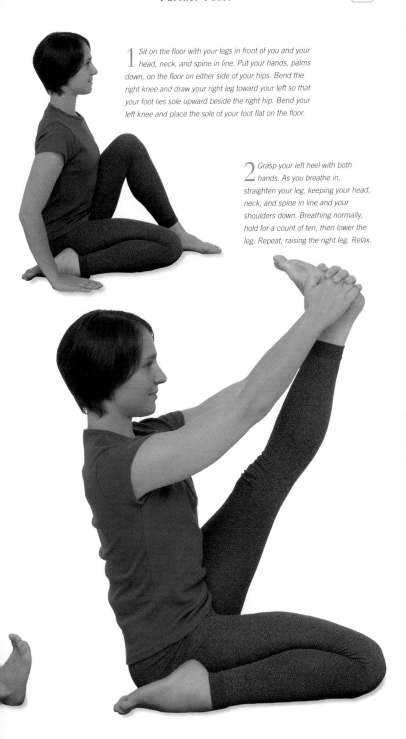

1 Sit on the floor with your legs in front of you and your head, neck, and spine in line. Put your hands, palms down, on the floor on either side of your hips. Bend the right knee and draw your right leg toward your left so that your foot lies sole upward beside the right hip. Bend left knee and place the sole of your foot flat on the floor.

2 Grasp your left heel with both hands. As you breathe in, straighten your leg, keeping your head, neck, and spine in line and your shoulders down. Breathing normally, hold for a count of ten, then lower the leg. Repeat, raising the right leg. Relax.

The Eagle Arms Pose

Most people's shoulders get very little exercise and are one of the first parts of the body to become tense and stiff when you are feeling stressed. This pose loosens the joints and strengthens the muscles in the shoulders, upper back, arms, and wrists, increasing circulation to these areas and opening up the chest. The full Eagle (*see pages 68–69*) is a standing pose in which both arms and legs are twisted. Practicing just the arm twist will make it easier to balance when holding the standing pose.

1 *Start in the* Classic Thunderbolt *(see page 51). While breathing in, stretch both arms out to the sides at shoulder level. As you breathe out, swing your arms forward to hug yourself, crossing your right upper arm over your left upper arm at chest level.*

2 *Raise your forearms to an upright position in front of your face, with your upper arms still crossed. Keep the backs of your hands together and point your fingers upward. Move your left hand slightly toward you and your right slightly away from you, sliding the palms together as flat as possible.*

3 *Keeping your shoulders down, your palms together, and your fingers pointing upward, raise your elbows to shoulder level and move them slightly away from your chest. Hold the position for a count of 20, then release your hands and shake them. Repeat, crossing your left upper arm over your right upper arm in Step 1.*

The Mermaid

In this seated pose, the trunk is gently rotated, which loosens tension in the upper back and stiffness in the spine, neck, and shoulders. You may prefer to practice this pose sitting on a foam block or folded rug, which helps to raise your pelvis and lever your trunk further round as you twist.

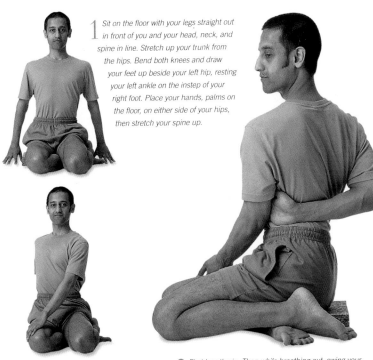

1 Sit on the floor with your legs straight out in front of you and your head, neck, and spine in line. Stretch up your trunk from the hips. Bend both knees and draw your feet up beside your left hip, resting your left ankle on the instep of your right foot. Place your hands, palms on the floor, on either side of your hips, then stretch your spine up.

2 While breathing out, turn your trunk from the hips to your right. Place your left hand on your right thigh and pull gently to rotate to the right, without jerking, and press your right hand down behind you. As you press down, lift and rotate your trunk a little further, but only as far as is comfortable.

3 First breathe in. Then while breathing out, swing your right arm behind you and clasp your left upper arm. Place the back of your left hand on the outside of your right thigh just above the knee. Turn your head to look over your left shoulder. Breathing normally, twist a little further for a count of ten. Keep your shoulders in line as you twist and don't let one rise higher than the other. Turn to face forward and straighten your legs to return to the starting position. Repeat, twisting to the left.

The Warrior Lunge

The back, shoulders, and neck all benefit from this version
of the Warrior pose, which is a little more demanding than the
version described earlier (*see pages 64–65*). As well as increasing
spinal flexibility and releasing muscular tension, it is also very
invigorating and creates a positive mental attitude. It is one
of the classic yoga poses described as "auspicious."

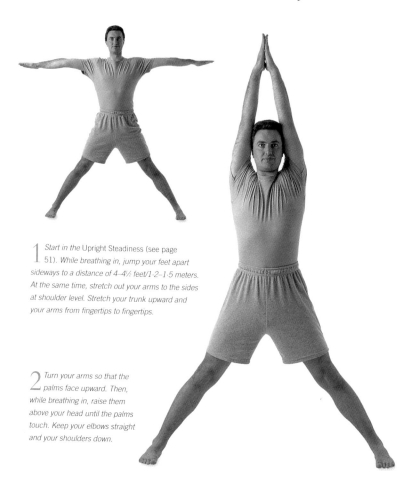

1 *Start in the* Upright Steadiness *(see page
51). While breathing in, jump your feet apart
sideways to a distance of 4–4½ feet/1·2–1·5 meters.
At the same time, stretch out your arms to the sides
at shoulder level. Stretch your trunk upward and
your arms from fingertips to fingertips.*

2 *Turn your arms so that the
palms face upward. Then,
while breathing in, raise them
above your head until the palms
touch. Keep your elbows straight
and your shoulders down.*

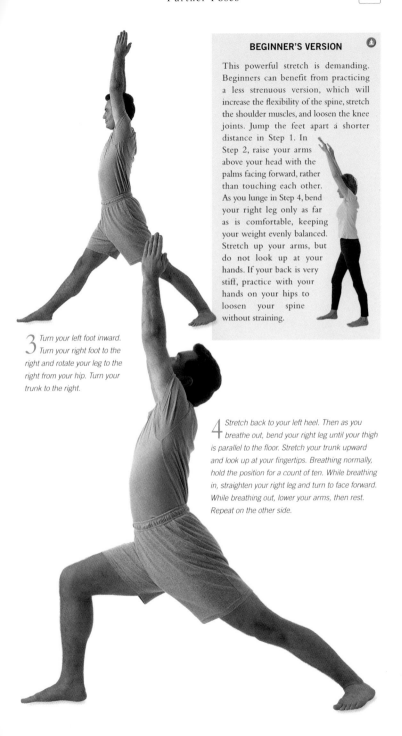

BEGINNER'S VERSION

This powerful stretch is demanding. Beginners can benefit from practicing a less strenuous version, which will increase the flexibility of the spine, stretch the shoulder muscles, and loosen the knee joints. Jump the feet apart a shorter distance in Step 1. In Step 2, raise your arms above your head with the palms facing forward, rather than touching each other. As you lunge in Step 4, bend your right leg only as far as is comfortable, keeping your weight evenly balanced. Stretch up your arms, but do not look up at your hands. If your back is very stiff, practice with your hands on your hips to loosen your spine without straining.

3 Turn your left foot inward. Turn your right foot to the right and rotate your leg to the right from your hip. Turn your trunk to the right.

4 Stretch back to your left heel. Then as you breathe out, bend your right leg until your thigh is parallel to the floor. Stretch your trunk upward and look up at your fingertips. Breathing normally, hold the position for a count of ten. While breathing in, straighten your right leg and turn to face forward. While breathing out, lower your arms, then rest. Repeat on the other side.

The Simple Warrior with Balance

Strength, stamina, coordination, and balance are all enhanced by this pose. It raises your energy levels and increases vitality. A full body stretch, it is particularly good for firming the buttocks. Advanced students can make this a continuation of the Warrior Lunge (*see pages 122–123*).

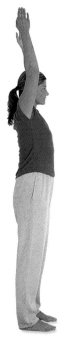 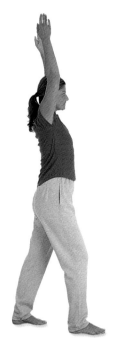 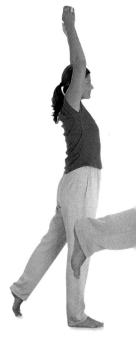

1 *Stand in the* Upright Steadiness (see page 51). *Breathing normally, raise your arms above your head, keeping your shoulders down. Place your palms together and straighten your elbows.*

2 *Step forward on to your right foot, keeping your head, neck, and spine in line, but transferring your weight to your right foot.*

3 *While breathing in deeply, extend your left leg behind you until it is straight, "locking" your right knee and keeping your head, neck, and spine in line. Breathe out.*

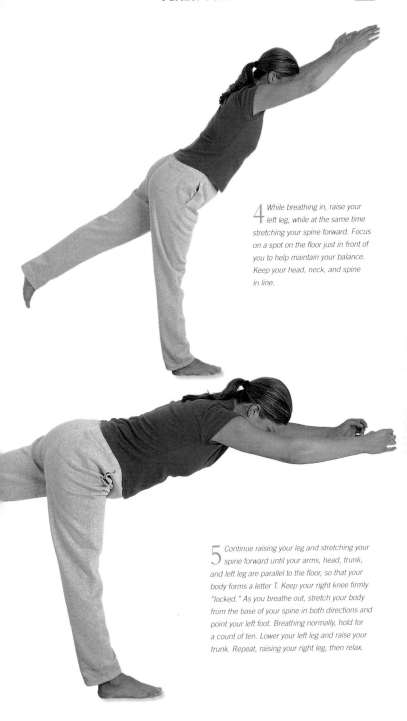

4 While breathing in, raise your left leg, while at the same time stretching your spine forward. Focus on a spot on the floor just in front of you to help maintain your balance. Keep your head, neck, and spine in line.

5 Continue raising your leg and stretching your spine forward until your arms, head, trunk, and left leg are parallel to the floor, so that your body forms a letter T. Keep your right knee firmly "locked." As you breathe out, stretch your body from the base of your spine in both directions and point your left foot. Breathing normally, hold for a count of ten. Lower your left leg and raise your trunk. Repeat, raising your right leg, then relax.

Wide Legs Posture

Prasarita Padottanasana combines the benefits of stretching
the muscles of the legs and pelvis with those of inverted poses.
It increases the flexibility of the hips, strengthens the hamstrings,
and gets rid of superfluous fat around the hips. It also increases
the blood supply to the head and face, which is why inverted
poses are said to increase both brains and beauty.

1 *Start in the* Upright Steadiness
(see page 51). *While breathing
in, jump your feet apart sideways to
a distance of about 5 feet/1.5 meters.
Place your hands on your hips and
turn both feet slightly inward. Keep
your head, neck, and spine in line.*

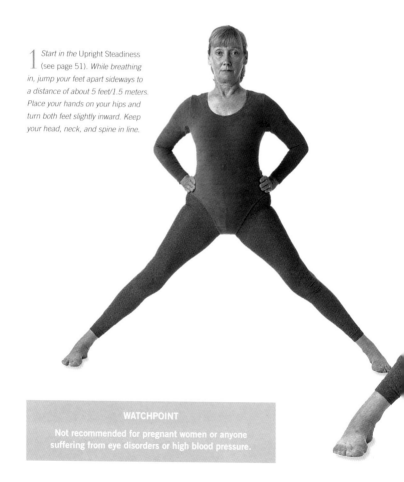

WATCHPOINT
Not recommended for pregnant women or anyone
suffering from eye disorders or high blood pressure.

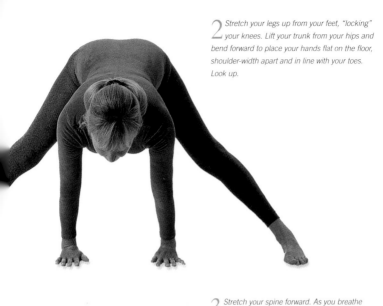

2 Stretch your legs up from your feet, "locking" your knees. Lift your trunk from your hips and bend forward to place your hands flat on the floor, shoulder-width apart and in line with your toes. Look up.

3 Stretch your spine forward. As you breathe out, bend your elbows and lower your head until the crown rests on the floor between your hands. Breathing normally, hold the position for a count of 15. Raise your head, then straighten your arms and stand up slowly. Breathe out and jump to bring your feet together.

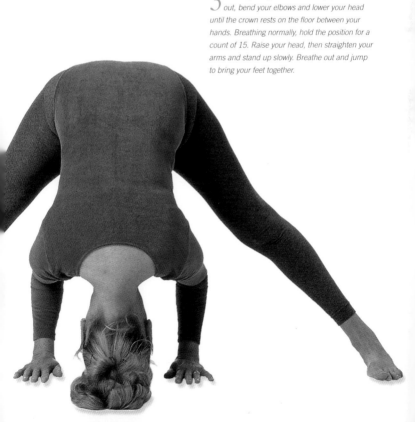

Lunge Twist

This pose increases the suppleness of the legs, waist, and back; tones the muscles of the shoulders and sides; builds stamina and strength; and improves balance. The strong rotation increases the flexibility of the spine and loosens the shoulder joints. This is a strenuous pose and you should stop immediately if it causes pain.

1 *Start in the* Classic Thunderbolt *(see page 51), then raise your hips until your thighs are at right angles to the floor and your arms are by your sides. Place your left foot flat on the floor in front of you, with your right hand, palm downward, resting on your thigh just above your knee. Place your left hand behind your right hip and then, by pulling on your left knee, twist to the left from your hips.*

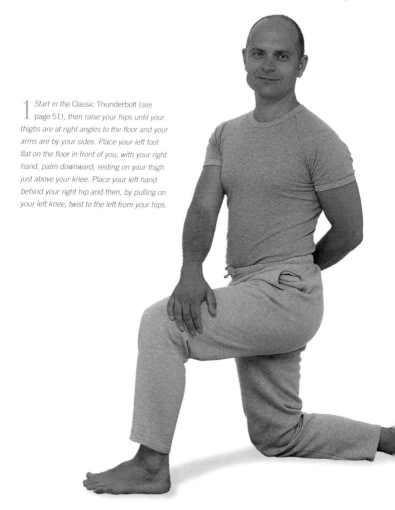

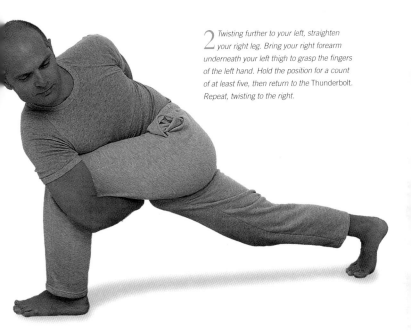

2 Twisting further to your left, straighten your right leg. Bring your right forearm underneath your left thigh to grasp the fingers of the left hand. Hold the position for a count of at least five, then return to the Thunderbolt. *Repeat, twisting to the right.*

DEEP LUNGE

This pose combines the muscle toning benefits of the lunge with the improvement in spinal flexibility of the twist. Stand with your feet wide apart and your head, neck, and spine in line. Clasp your hands behind your back. While breathing out, bend forward and bend your right knee. Lower your forehead as close to your right foot as possible, keeping your hands clasped behind your back. Hold the position for a count of at least five, then return to the starting position. Repeat, bending to the left. Do not force yourself to bend or twist further than is comfortable—stop if the pose causes any pain.

The Bow

Dhanurasana is an extreme stretch that strengthens and tones the muscles of the back and front of the body; loosens the spine, hips, and shoulder joints; massages the abdominal organs; and stimulates the circulation. If you find the full pose difficult, practice only the first two steps until your body is more supple.

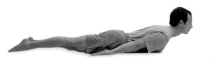

1 Lie prone on the floor with your arms by your sides and your legs slightly apart. When you are first learning the pose, it is easier if you spread your knees well apart. Raise your legs slightly and stretch them back.

2 Bend your knees and bring your heels back close to your bottom, keeping your thighs stretched back. Grasp your ankles, not your feet, with your hands. Do not point your toes. Keeping your elbows straight, pull on your ankle, and lift your thighs and chest off the floor. Authorities differ as to whether you should breathe in, breathe out, or breathe how you like as you pull on your ankles. It is quite hard to concentrate on your breathing in this pose—breathing normally is probably the best option.

3 Raise your head a little more, looking forward, and lift your shins higher, so that your body is resting entirely on your abdomen. Hold the pose for a count of ten. Release your ankles, then lower your legs and trunk to the floor. Relax before repeating.

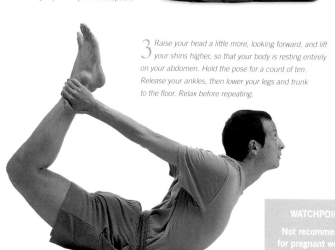

WATCHPOINT
Not recommended for pregnant women.

The Camel

Ustrasana is a stretch that strengthens the spine and tones the neck, waist, and tummy—the perfect counter to poor posture. In the full pose, the head is thrown back and the spine bent in a single movement. When learning this less demanding version, you may find it easier to spread your knees and feet further apart.

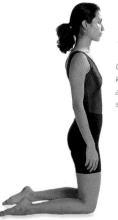

1 *Start in the* Classic Thunderbolt *(see page 51). While breathing in, lift your hips and trunk so you are kneeling upright with your head, neck, and spine in line and hands by your sides. Do not move your legs or feet.*

2 *Lean back, keeping your shoulders down and letting your hands dangle. When you have reached a comfortable stable position, stretch back with your right hand and rest your fingers on your right heel. If this is too difficult, practice by placing your hand on the floor behind your foot.*

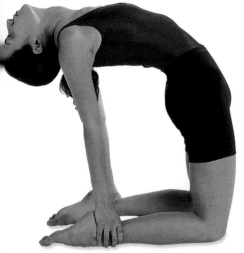

3 *Let your head drop back and reach down to rest the fingers of your left hand on your left heel or, if necessary, rest your hand on the floor behind your left foot. Breathing normally, hold the position for a count of ten. While breathing in, lift your hands and raise your head, then return to the* Thunderbolt.

The Wheel

Chakrasana stretches and strengthens the muscles of the
abdomen and loosens the spine. It also strengthens the ankles
and wrists, stimulates the circulation, and is thought to alleviate
some throat problems. This pose helps to build stamina and
creates a positive mental attitude. It does require reasonable
flexibility and strength, but is not so daunting as it might at
first appear. Advanced students can learn to achieve this
posture from standing, but this requires considerable spinal
strength and flexibility and should be practiced under
the guidance of a teacher.

1 *Lie flat on your back with your knees bent and slightly apart and
the soles of your feet flat on the floor near your bottom. When you
are learning this pose, it may help to have your legs and feet further
apart. Place the palms of your hands flat on the floor beside your head
with your elbows pointing upward. Keeping your feet flat on the floor
and parallel to each other, lift your hips off the floor, followed by your
trunk, then your head, so that only the soles of your feet, the crown of
your head, and your palms remain on the floor.*

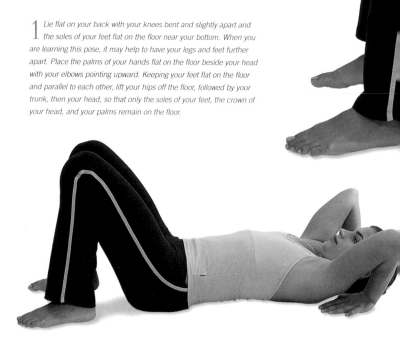

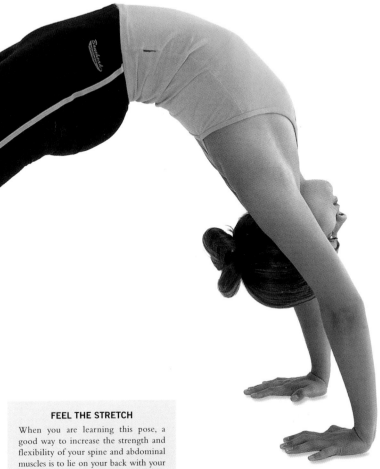

FEEL THE STRETCH

When you are learning this pose, a good way to increase the strength and flexibility of your spine and abdominal muscles is to lie on your back with your head, neck, and spine in line, your arms by your sides, your knees bent and slightly apart, and the soles of your feet flat on the floor near your bottom. Grasp your left ankle with your left hand and your right ankle with your right hand. Then, keeping your feet, head, and shoulders on the floor, lift your hips and chest as high as possible. You should be able to feel the stretch in your upper back, chest, and hips. Breathing deeply, hold for a count of ten, then lower your hips and trunk and rest. Repeat several times. Practice this, for weeks if necessary, until you feel confident about trying the complete pose.

2 *While breathing in, straighten your elbows and raise your hips and chest as high as possible, letting your head drop back. Keep the soles of your feet flat on the floor. Breathing normally, hold the position for at least a count of five. Gently lower your body and rest.*

The Half Moon

The *Ardha Chandrasana* tones the muscles and joints of the legs and hips; strengthens the spine; and gets rid of superfluous fat around the waist. It is also beneficial to the digestive and nervous systems. It is an excellent pose to practice if you suffer from weak knees or ankles, and improves balance.

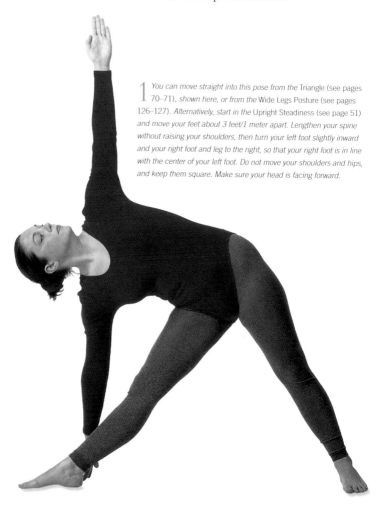

1 *You can move straight into this pose from the* Triangle *(see pages 70–71), shown here, or from the* Wide Legs Posture *(see pages 126–127). Alternatively, start in the* Upright Steadiness *(see page 51) and move your feet about 3 feet/1 meter apart. Lengthen your spine without raising your shoulders, then turn your left foot slightly inward and your right foot and leg to the right, so that your right foot is in line with the center of your left foot. Do not move your shoulders and hips, and keep them square. Make sure your head is facing forward.*

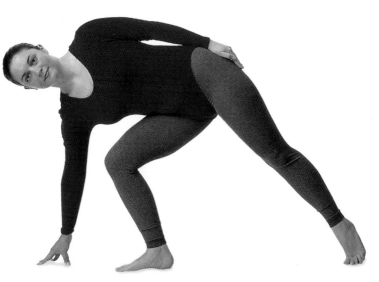

2 While breathing out, bend your right leg, then lean
over to the right from your hips and place your
right hand, palm downward, flat on the floor and about
12 inches/30 cm in front of your right foot. Keep your
hips and shoulders square. If you find it too difficult
to rest your palm on the floor, rest the tips of your fingers.
Rest your left arm along your side.

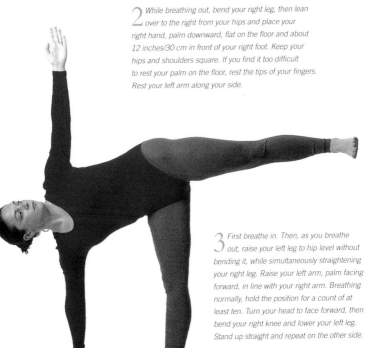

3 First breathe in. Then, as you breathe
out, raise your left leg to hip level without
bending it, while simultaneously straightening
your right leg. Raise your left arm, palm facing
forward, in line with your right arm. Breathing
normally, hold the position for a count of at
least ten. Turn your head to face forward, then
bend your right knee and lower your left leg.
Stand up straight and repeat on the other side.

The Lord of the Dance

Natarajasana is a balancing pose, most usually seen with one leg raised and bent in front of the body. B. K. S. Iyengar developed a variation in which the leg is raised behind the body and the toe grasped between the thumb and forefinger. The elbow and shoulder of that arm are then rotated over the head to pull the foot up toward the head. It is a very advanced pose, requiring great flexibility and superb balance. This is a slightly less demanding version of Iyengar's variation, which you can learn in stages.

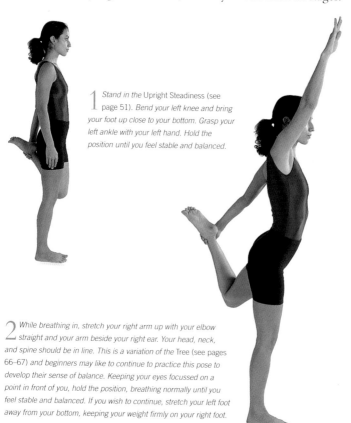

1 *Stand in the* Upright Steadiness (see page 51). *Bend your left knee and bring your foot up close to your bottom. Grasp your left ankle with your left hand. Hold the position until you feel stable and balanced.*

2 *While breathing in, stretch your right arm up with your elbow straight and your arm beside your right ear. Your head, neck, and spine should be in line. This is a variation of the* Tree *(see pages 66–67) and beginners may like to continue to practice this pose to develop their sense of balance. Keeping your eyes focussed on a point in front of you, hold the position, breathing normally until you feel stable and balanced. If you wish to continue, stretch your left foot away from your bottom, keeping your weight firmly on your right foot.*

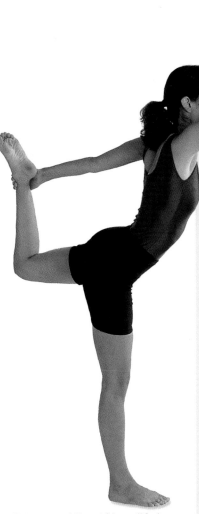

HELPFUL HINTS

Learning this pose takes time and it is not uncommon to develop a wobble just as you are progressing to the next step, or even to lose hold of your ankle. To help maintain your balance, keep your eyes focussed on a point just in front of you. As you begin to shift your weight forward in Step 3, transfer your focus to a point on the floor just in front of you. If your ankle constantly slips out of your grasp, check that you are holding your ankle and not the top of your foot. You can also practice holding a belt tied around your foot so that you can concentrate on achieving perfect balance. Aligning your body properly is crucial. Keep your weight evenly and firmly on your supporting leg, with your knee pressed back. Do not turn your hips toward your bent leg, twist your head to one side, or let your raised arm drift away from your ear. When concentrating on a new and demanding pose, it is very common to hold your breath—don't. When completing Step 3 and shifting your weight forward, be aware of your balance and don't force yourself further than you can manage, or you may topple over.

3 Straighten and lift your left knee, still firmly grasping your ankle. You are aiming to have your left thigh parallel with the floor, but do not strain your muscles. When you can do this and retain your balance, breathe normally and slowly shift your weight forward, keeping your right arm beside your ear. Stop while you are still stable and balanced, and hold the position for as long as you feel stable and comfortable. With practice, you should be able to shift your weight forward so that your right arm, chest, and left thigh are all parallel to the ground, with your head, neck, and spine in line. Finally, return to an upright position and lower your leg. Relax, then repeat on the other side.

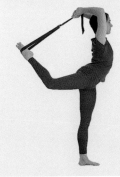

The Half Lotus Bend

Many of the postures learned by beginners can also be done in the Half Lotus by more advanced students. This forward stretch, *Ardha-Padmottanasana*, strengthens and tones the legs and hips, and helps remove any superfluous fat from the waistline. It improves balance and, because the abdominal organs are massaged, it aids digestion.

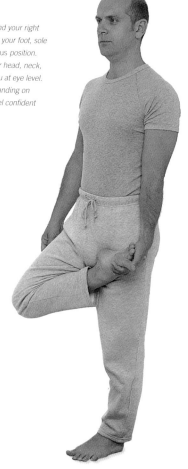

1 *Stand in the* Upright Steadiness *(see page 51). Bend your right knee and grasp your foot with your left hand. Place your foot, sole facing upward, high up on your left thigh in the* Half Lotus *position. Make sure that your left knee is "locked" and keep your head, neck, and spine in line. Fix your gaze on a point in front of you at eye level. Before moving on to the next step, practice this one, standing on alternate legs until you can manage it easily and you feel confident that you are securely balanced.*

THE VERSATILE HALF LOTUS

If you don't feel very confident about the forward bend and are worried about overbalancing, practice other balances in *Half Lotus* to improve your steadiness. For *Half Lotus Tree*, stand in the *Upright Steadiness (see page 51)*. Bend your right knee and grasp your foot with your left hand. Place your foot, sole facing upward, high up on your left thigh in the *Half Lotus* position. Keep your head, neck, and spine in line and "lock" your left knee. When you feel firmly balanced, place your hands, palms together, at chest height in the *Prayer* position *(see page 58)*. Try not to waver or wobble, and focus on a point in front of you at eye level. When you feel firmly balanced, keeping your palms together, straighten your arms above your head. Breathing normally, hold the pose for as long as is comfortable. Lower your arms and leg. Repeat, bending your left leg.

2 Breathing out, bend forward to place the palm of your left hand flat on the floor in front of your left foot and the palm of your right hand flat on the floor in front of your right foot. Breathing normally, hold for a count of ten, then raise your trunk and lower your leg. Repeat on the other side. With practice, you may be able to manage the full pose, putting the palms of your hands flat on the floor beside and in line with their respective feet, and placing your face against your left knee.

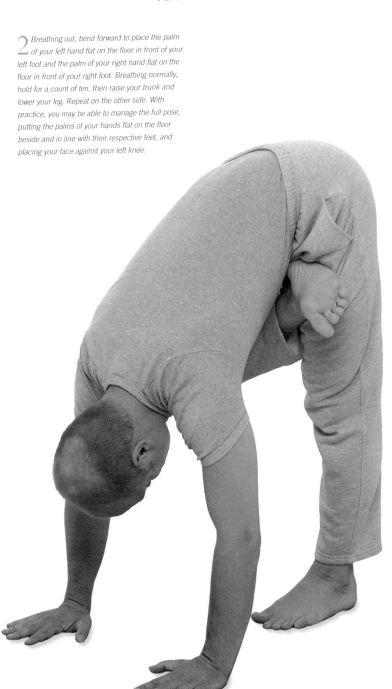

The Half Lotus in Dog

This is another pose that is familiar to beginners and which more advanced students can practice in Half Lotus. It has all the benefit of the basic *Dog* pose (*see pages 80–81*) and also increases the flexibility of the hips and improves balance.

Kneel on all fours, with your hands beneath your shoulders and pointing slightly inward and your thighs vertical and slightly apart. Your back, neck, and head should be in line and parallel to the floor. Place your right foot, sole upward, high up on your left thigh in the *Half Lotus* position. As you breathe in, raise your hips, pushing down on the palms of your hands, while straightening your left leg. Drop your head so that it is in line with your spine. Breathing normally, hold for a count of ten. Return to kneeling on all fours and repeat with your left foot placed on your right thigh.

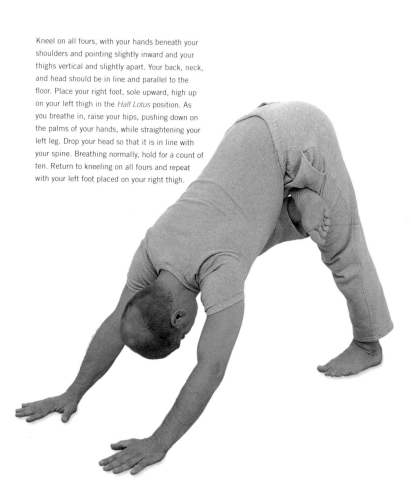

The Side Dog

This pose begins in the position familiar as a push-up.
The aim, however, is not to perform repetitions, but to hold
the pose correctly. It improves posture and balance; stimulates the
circulation; and tones the muscles of the arms, shoulders, back, and
legs. Its name is a mystery—no dog has ever been seen to do this.

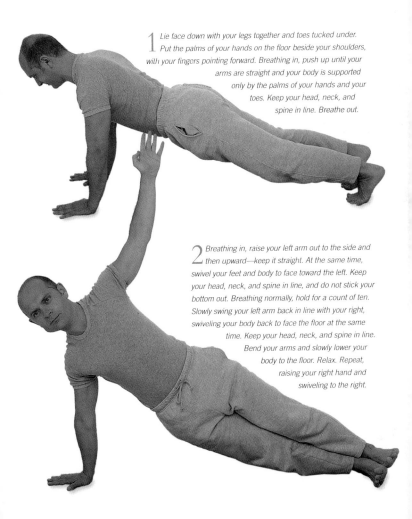

1 *Lie face down with your legs together and toes tucked under. Put the palms of your hands on the floor beside your shoulders, with your fingers pointing forward. Breathing in, push up until your arms are straight and your body is supported only by the palms of your hands and your toes. Keep your head, neck, and spine in line. Breathe out.*

2 *Breathing in, raise your left arm out to the side and then upward—keep it straight. At the same time, swivel your feet and body to face toward the left. Keep your head, neck, and spine in line, and do not stick your bottom out. Breathing normally, hold for a count of ten. Slowly swing your left arm back in line with your right, swiveling your body back to face the floor at the same time. Keep your head, neck, and spine in line. Bend your arms and slowly lower your body to the floor. Relax. Repeat, raising your right hand and swiveling to the right.*

Squatting Balances

These postures improve both balance and concentration, and strengthen the feet, knees, and thighs. They can help alleviate stiffness and aches in the lower back, especially if you have been on your feet all day. Before you move on to Step 3, practice the tiptoe squatting in Steps 1 and 2 until you feel comfortable holding the position for a count of at least ten.

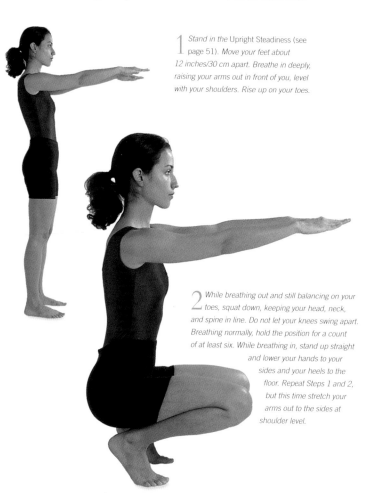

1 *Stand in the* Upright Steadiness *(see page 51). Move your feet about 12 inches/30 cm apart. Breathe in deeply, raising your arms out in front of you, level with your shoulders. Rise up on your toes.*

2 *While breathing out and still balancing on your toes, squat down, keeping your head, neck, and spine in line. Do not let your knees swing apart. Breathing normally, hold the position for a count of at least six. While breathing in, stand up straight and lower your hands to your sides and your heels to the floor. Repeat Steps 1 and 2, but this time stretch your arms out to the sides at shoulder level.*

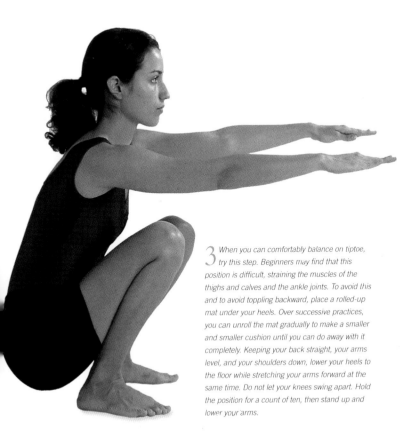

3 When you can comfortably balance on tiptoe, try this step. Beginners may find that this position is difficult, straining the muscles of the thighs and calves and the ankle joints. To avoid this and to avoid toppling backward, place a rolled-up mat under your heels. Over successive practices, you can unroll the mat gradually to make a smaller and smaller cushion until you can do away with it completely. Keeping your back straight, your arms level, and your shoulders down, lower your heels to the floor while stretching your arms forward at the same time. Do not let your knees swing apart. Hold the position for a count of ten, then stand up and lower your arms.

HARDER THAN IT LOOKS

Balancing in a squat initially requires more concentration and equilibrium than you might think. When you feel comfortable and balanced in the basic position shown here, and no longer require a rolled-up rug as a cushion to assist you, try achieving the same pose starting with your feet together. Then try to do it with your hands in the *Prayer* position (*see page 58*) in front of you and, eventually, try it with your hands in the prayer position behind your back (*see page 102*).

An alternative position, which offers the same benefits and also tones the abdomen and pelvis, is the *Single-Foot Squatting Balance*. Stand in the *Upright Steadiness* (*see page 51*). While breathing in deeply, rise up on your toes. As you breathe out, bend your knees and squat down, still balancing on your toes. Press your fingertips on the floor to steady yourself. Keeping your head, neck, and spine in line, stretch out your right leg straight in front of you with the toes pointing upward. Hold the position for a count of at least five, then bend your right knee, placing your right foot next to your left. While breathing in, stand up and lower your heels. Repeat, extending your left leg. When you are comfortable and stable in this position, you can raise your arms in front of you, parallel to the floor and at shoulder height before holding the balance.

The Crane

Bakasana brings balance to both mind and body, because it demands a high level of concentration. It strengthens the shoulders, arms, and wrists; loosens the joints of the upper body; and massages the abdominal organs.

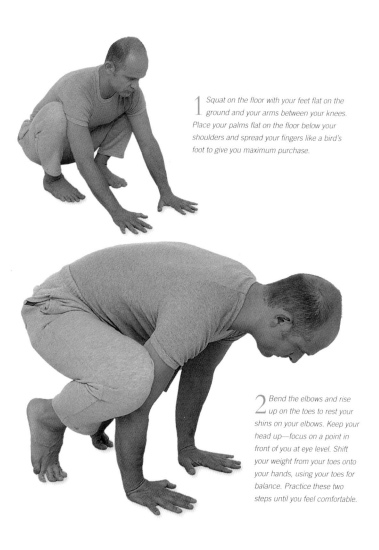

1 Squat on the floor with your feet flat on the ground and your arms between your knees. Place your palms flat on the floor below your shoulders and spread your fingers like a bird's foot to give you maximum purchase.

2 Bend the elbows and rise up on the toes to rest your shins on your elbows. Keep your head up—focus on a point in front of you at eye level. Shift your weight from your toes onto your hands, using your toes for balance. Practice these two steps until you feel comfortable.

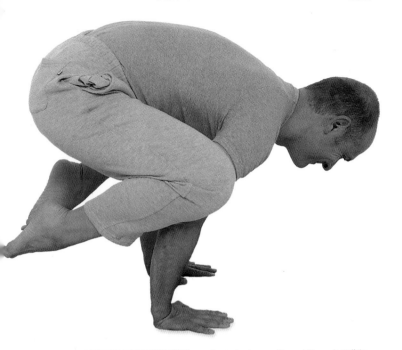

THE INVERTED CROW

In this more advanced posture, the knees are placed on the upper arms in Step 2. It looks more difficult than it is. Kneel down and place the palms of your hands on the floor, shoulder-width apart, with your fingers pointing forward and spread apart. Place the top of your head on the floor and "kneel" on your upper arms. Like any other version of the headstand, you should learn this pose under the supervision of a qualified teacher.

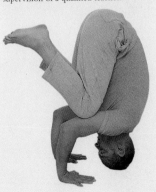

3 *Slowly raise your hips and lift your feet off the ground, keeping your head up. When learning this pose, you may find it easier to lift one foot followed by the other, rather than the two together. Hold the position for as long as is comfortable.*

The Little Boat

This pose limbers the legs and hips; relieves tension in the
back and shoulders; and increases spinal flexibility. It gently
massages the abdominal organs, which benefits the digestive
system and has an energizing effect.

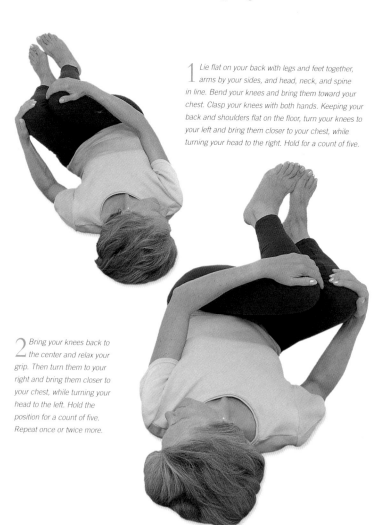

1 Lie flat on your back with legs and feet together,
arms by your sides, and head, neck, and spine
in line. Bend your knees and bring them toward your
chest. Clasp your knees with both hands. Keeping your
back and shoulders flat on the floor, turn your knees to
your left and bring them closer to your chest, while
turning your head to the right. Hold for a count of five.

2 Bring your knees back to
the center and relax your
grip. Then turn them to your
right and bring them closer to
your chest, while turning your
head to the left. Hold the
position for a count of five.
Repeat once or twice more.

The Boat Poses

Both these poses, the Half Boat (*Ardha Navasana*) and the Boat
with Oars (*Navasana*), strengthen the muscles of the back and
abdomen and benefit the liver, spleen, gall bladder, and nervous
system. They also increase your balance and concentration.

The Half Boat

1 *Sit on the floor with your
legs in front of you and your
head, neck, and spine in line.
Place your hands, palms on the
floor, on either side of your hips.
Stretch up your trunk from the
hips. Interlace your fingers and
clasp them behind your head
While breathing in, raise your
trunk from your hips.*

2 *While breathing out, lean your
trunk backward toward the floor,
while raising your legs until your toes
are level with your eyes. Don't point
your toes. Breathing quickly, hold the
position for a count of at least five.
Lower your legs, then sit up and rest.*

Boat with Oars

1 *Sit on the floor with your legs straight out in front
of you and your head, neck, and spine in line.
Place your hands, palms on the floor, on either side
of your hips. Stretch up your trunk from the hips.
While breathing out, lean your trunk backward toward
the floor, while raising your legs, feet together, until
your toes are higher than your head. Keep your legs
straight, but don't point your toes.*

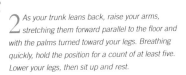

2 *As your trunk leans back, raise your arms,
stretching them forward parallel to the floor and
with the palms turned toward your legs. Breathing
quickly, hold the position for a count of at least five.
Lower your legs, then sit up and rest.*

The Pose of Tranquillity

This pose has acquired its name because it is surprisingly relaxing—it's good to do just before bedtime if you suffer from insomnia. It also strengthens the abdominal muscles and stretches the spine and back muscles. Beginners can practice it over time and in easy stages to increase muscular control, thus ensuring that the final pose is completed in a smooth, flowing movement.

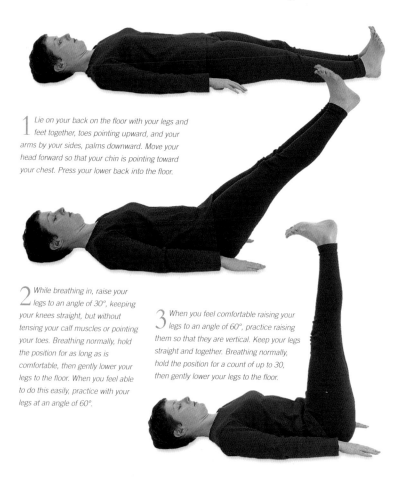

1 Lie on your back on the floor with your legs and feet together, toes pointing upward, and your arms by your sides, palms downward. Move your head forward so that your chin is pointing toward your chest. Press your lower back into the floor.

2 While breathing in, raise your legs to an angle of 30°, keeping your knees straight, but without tensing your calf muscles or pointing your toes. Breathing normally, hold the position for as long as is comfortable, then gently lower your legs to the floor. When you feel able to do this easily, practice with your legs at an angle of 60°.

3 When you feel comfortable raising your legs to an angle of 60°, practice raising them so that they are vertical. Keep your legs straight and together. Breathing normally, hold the position for a count of up to 30, then gently lower your legs to the floor.

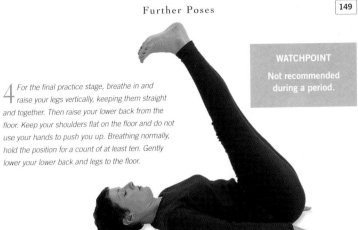

4 For the final practice stage, breathe in and raise your legs vertically, keeping them straight and together. Then raise your lower back from the floor. Keep your shoulders flat on the floor and do not use your hands to push you up. Breathing normally, hold the position for a count of at least ten. Gently lower your lower back and legs to the floor.

WATCHPOINT

Not recommended during a period.

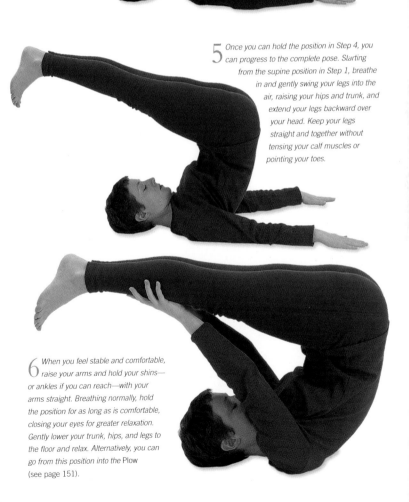

5 Once you can hold the position in Step 4, you can progress to the complete pose. Starting from the supine position in Step 1, breathe in and gently swing your legs into the air, raising your hips and trunk, and extend your legs backward over your head. Keep your legs straight and together without tensing your calf muscles or pointing your toes.

6 When you feel stable and comfortable, raise your arms and hold your shins— or ankles if you can reach—with your arms straight. Breathing normally, hold the position for as long as is comfortable, closing your eyes for greater relaxation. Gently lower your trunk, hips, and legs to the floor and relax. Alternatively, you can go from this position into the Plow (see page 151).

Shoulder Stand

This pose benefits the entire body—its name, *Sarvangasana*, means "complete body." It is also known in English as the All Body posture or Candle pose. It stretches the spine; benefits the heart and lungs; regulates the metabolism; and relieves varicose veins. Like all inverted postures, it is very relaxing.

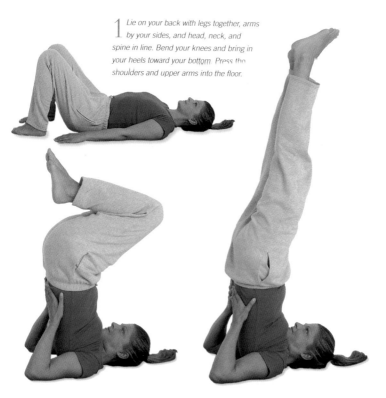

1 Lie on your back with legs together, arms by your sides, and head, neck, and spine in line. Bend your knees and bring in your heels toward your bottom. Press the shoulders and upper arms into the floor.

2 Breathe in. Press your arms down and raise the legs and hips to bring your bent knees over your head—keep the back straight. Bend your elbows to put your hands on each side of the spine, fingers pointing at your spine, to support the back.

3 Keeping your legs together, straighten until the feet are above the shoulders. Breathe normally, holding for a count of at least 30. Lower the feet to an angle of 45° and put your hands on the floor. Unroll slowly. Relax in the Corpse (see page 60).

The Plow

This extreme forward bend stretches the whole body; strengthens the back; increases the flexibility of the spine in both back and neck; and massages the internal organs. The version shown here is the Supported Plow.

LEARNING THE PLOW

To practice with a chair, start from Step 2 or Step 3 of the *Shoulder Stand*. From Step 2, straighten your legs and place your feet on the seat of the chair, resting on your toes. From Step 3, lower your feet over your head until your toes are resting on the chair. In both cases, hold for a count of at least 30.

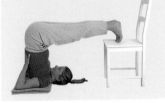

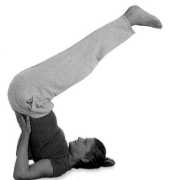

1 *Start from the* Shoulder Stand *(see opposite). Breathing out and keeping the legs together and knees straight, slowly lower your feet toward the floor behind your head. Do not force them lower than is comfortable. Practice until your spine becomes more flexible and your back muscles are stronger.*

2 *Bring your toes to the floor, keeping your legs straight. Breathing normally, hold for a count of at least 30. Intermediate students may like to complete the full pose first: place your hands, flat on the ground and arms parallel, behind your back, and tuck in your toes and lower your heels. Bend your knees and return to the* Shoulder Stand *position, then lower your feet to an angle of 45° and place your hands flat on the floor. Unroll slowly and relax in the* Corpse *(see page 60).*

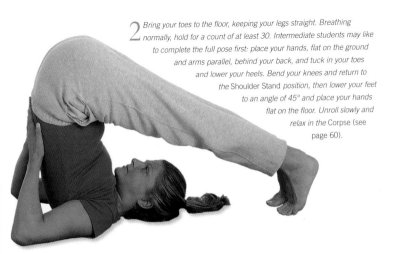

Shoulder Stand Variations

The Shoulder Stand, Plow, and Bridge are often grouped in a cycle. Try the following sequence: Shoulder Stand, Half Plow, Shoulder Stand, Plow or Wide-Legged Plow, Shoulder Stand, Bridge, Raised Leg Bridge, Shoulder Stand, Corpse.

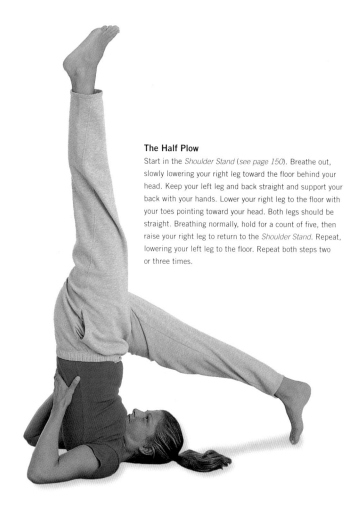

The Half Plow

Start in the *Shoulder Stand* (*see page 150*). Breathe out, slowly lowering your right leg toward the floor behind your head. Keep your left leg and back straight and support your back with your hands. Lower your right leg to the floor with your toes pointing toward your head. Both legs should be straight. Breathing normally, hold for a count of five, then raise your right leg to return to the *Shoulder Stand*. Repeat, lowering your left leg to the floor. Repeat both steps two or three times.

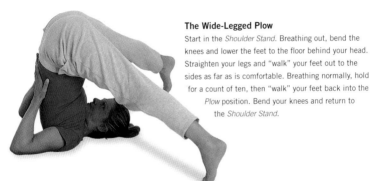

The Wide-Legged Plow

Start in the *Shoulder Stand*. Breathing out, bend the knees and lower the feet to the floor behind your head. Straighten your legs and "walk" your feet out to the sides as far as is comfortable. Breathing normally, hold for a count of ten, then "walk" your feet back into the *Plow* position. Bend your knees and return to the *Shoulder Stand*.

The Bridge

This is an alternative way for advanced students to come into the Bridge. Start in the *Shoulder Stand* and bend both knees. Slowly lower both feet to the floor behind your back with one foot leading. Do not move your hands or alter their position. Place both feet parallel and flat on the floor and raise your hips as high as possible. Breathing normally, hold for a count of 30.

The Raised Leg Bridge

Start in the *Bridge*. Breathing in and keeping your left foot on the floor, raise your right leg, bringing your foot toward the ceiling. Keep your right leg straight and bring it toward your head as far as possible. Do not let your hips drop. Hold for a count of ten, then lower your right leg and bend your knee to place your foot on the floor parallel with your left foot. Repeat, raising your left leg, then return to the *Shoulder Stand* without moving the position of your hands.

Headstand

The Headstand, *Sirsasna*, has so many benefits that it is known as the "King of Asanas." The reversal of gravity rests the heart, while increasing circulation to the brain, nervous system, scalp, and face. Many internal organs are toned, and it is helpful for sufferers of varicose veins or piles. Learn it in stages—quarter, half, and full—and ideally under the guidance of a teacher. Always come out of the position slowly and rest in the Child for a few minutes, and then the Corpse to avoid dizziness.

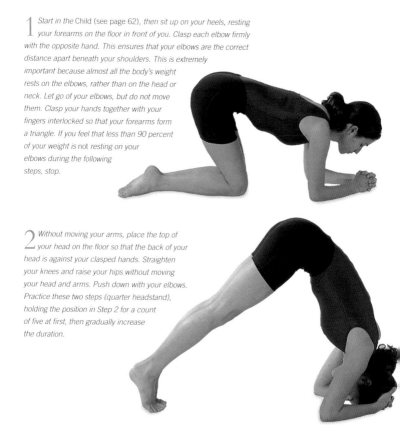

1 *Start in the Child (see page 62), then sit up on your heels, resting your forearms on the floor in front of you. Clasp each elbow firmly with the opposite hand. This ensures that your elbows are the correct distance apart beneath your shoulders. This is extremely important because almost all the body's weight rests on the elbows, rather than on the head or neck. Let go of your elbows, but do not move them. Clasp your hands together with your fingers interlocked so that your forearms form a triangle. If you feel that less than 90 percent of your weight is not resting on your elbows during the following steps, stop.*

2 *Without moving your arms, place the top of your head on the floor so that the back of your head is against your clasped hands. Straighten your knees and raise your hips without moving your head and arms. Push down with your elbows. Practice these two steps (quarter headstand), holding the position in Step 2 for a count of five at first, then gradually increase the duration.*

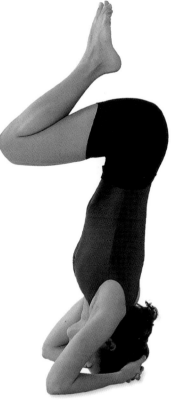

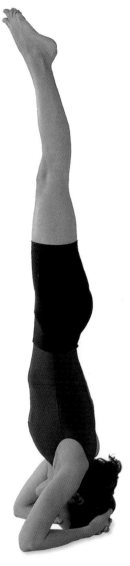

3 Keeping your hips up and your weight on your elbows, "walk" your feet toward your face. As you do so, your back will straighten and your hips will move up over your head. Bend your knees and lift your feet off the floor, bringing your heels smoothly up toward your bottom and tucking your knees toward your chest. Most of your weight should be on your elbows. Practice these three steps (half headstand), holding the position in Step 3 for a count of five at first, then gradually increasing the duration until you can hold it comfortably for a count of at least 30. From the half headstand, gradually raise your knees until they are pointing upward and your heels are pointing toward your bottom.

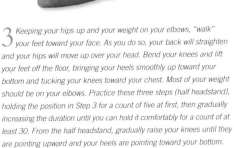

4 Gradually straighten your knees, bringing your feet up toward the ceiling, keeping your legs together, but without pointing your toes. Almost all your weight should be on your elbows and your body should be in a straight line from your heels to your head. Breathing normally, hold the position for a count of at least ten, very gradually building up the duration—do not let yourself become tired and wobbly. Bend your knees and lower your hips, then bring your feet to the floor. Sit back on your heels and rest in the Child.

Elbow Stand

This is an alternative version of the *Headstand (see page 154)*.
It should be learned under the supervision of a qualified
teacher to avoid risk of injury.

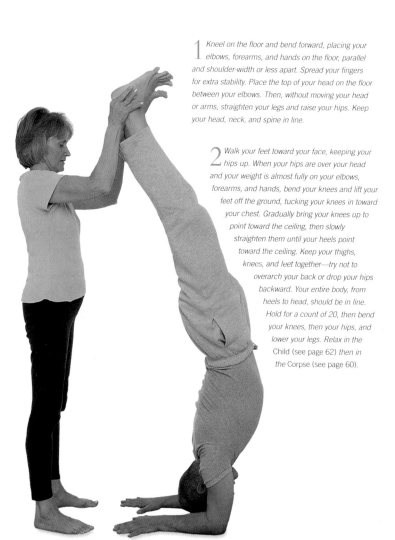

1 Kneel on the floor and bend forward, placing your
elbows, forearms, and hands on the floor, parallel
and shoulder-width or less apart. Spread your fingers
for extra stability. Place the top of your head on the floor
between your elbows. Then, without moving your head
or arms, straighten your legs and raise your hips. Keep
your head, neck, and spine in line.

2 Walk your feet toward your face, keeping your
hips up. When your hips are over your head
and your weight is almost fully on your elbows,
forearms, and hands, bend your knees and lift your
feet off the ground, tucking your knees in toward
your chest. Gradually bring your knees up to
point toward the ceiling, then slowly
straighten them until your heels point
toward the ceiling. Keep your thighs,
knees, and feet together—try not to
overarch your back or drop your hips
backward. Your entire body, from
heels to head, should be in line.
Hold for a count of 20, then bend
your knees, then your hips, and
lower your legs. Relax in the
Child (see page 62) then in
the Corpse (see page 60).

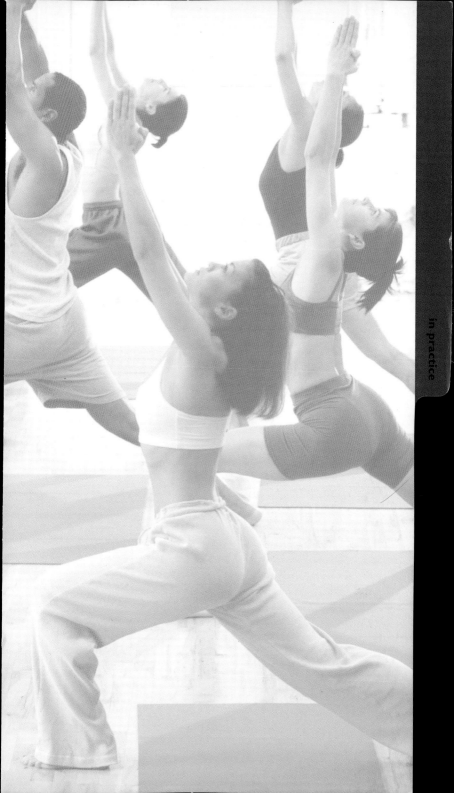

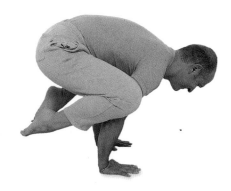

Yoga in Practice

The following six programs are simply suggestions and you may prefer your own routine. All the poses are either for beginners or are intermediate, and you should feel free to substitute a similar pose for the one suggested. The successive programs include increasingly advanced poses, but there is no timetable. Feeling confident in basic poses will benefit you far more than attempting something that is beyond your body's current capacity, which could also cause injury. Yoga is a pathway of discovery about both your body and your mind, and at the end of a yoga program, you should feel refreshed and re-energized. Above all, it should be a pleasure, not a chore.

Practicing Yoga

There are no instant results with yoga, but there are long-term benefits to be derived from regular practice. Try to set aside a regular time, but don't be too ambitious. Start with a fairly short session (about 30 minutes, once a week), then gradually build up your practice—if not every day, perhaps two or three times a week. You may also want to make the session longer, but don't carry on until you feel exhausted. It is better to practice just a few poses properly and smoothly than to drive yourself to perform twice as many and end up doing them half as well. The programs in this chapter have been designed in two halves, so if you complete the first seven postures, you can be confident that your practice is balanced. Absolute beginners may prefer to start with even fewer postures— one or two is fine. Don't rush through your yoga program as if it is just one more thing to tick off the list in a busy life. Yoga is not a competition.

You should always begin and end with a few minutes of relaxation and you can also relax between poses. The most popular pose for this is the *Corpse (see page 60)*, but the *Rescue Pose (see page 61)* is also good. Don't neglect warm-up exercises to loosen joints and muscles.

Your program should be balanced, so that a backward bend is countered by a forward bend, for example. If you want to work on a particular pose, either because you are learning it or because you want to concentrate on strengthening

You should always relax before starting your program, as well as at the end. This helps to focus your mind so that you are better able to concentrate fully on the poses.

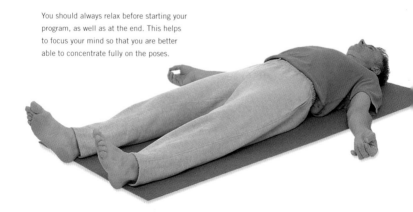

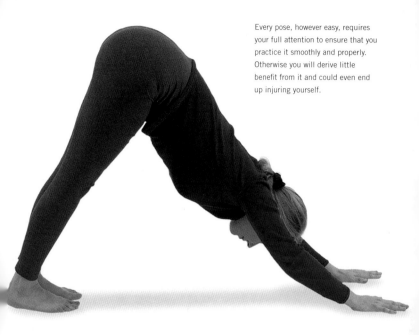

Every pose, however easy, requires your full attention to ensure that you practice it smoothly and properly. Otherwise you will derive little benefit from it and could even end up injuring yourself.

particular muscles or joints, do leave some time for some other poses as well. Remember, too, that if you have completed a posture which twists the spine to the right, for example, you should then repeat it twisting to the left. The programs in this chapter all include stretches, forward and backward bends, spinal twists, sitting or kneeling, limbering the legs, and an inverted pose. However, before you follow any of them or plan your own program, check the list of contraindications on pages 36–37 and the hints on page 172.

Make sure you have balance in everything. So always counter a forward bend, such as the *Dog* (*see pages 80–81*) shown above, with a backward bend, such as the *Half Locust* (*see page 77*). Similarly, stretches or twists to the right should be followed by the same movement to the left.

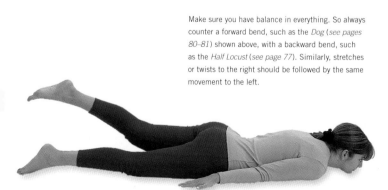

Program 1

Although the poses suggested here will be within the scope
of most beginners after a few months' practice, only you know
your own body's capacity, so never force yourself into a position
that causes discomfort or pain. The first seven poses—the *Palm
Tree*, the *Simple Forward Bend*, the *Cobra*, the *Simple Spinal Twist*,
the *Hero*, the *Squatting Balances*, and the *Hare*—complete a
sequence. If you wish to continue, you can either repeat this
sequence or continue with the *Triangle*, the *Cat*, the *Simple Sage*,
the *Cobbler*, the *Powerful Pose*, the *Pose of Tranquillity*, and the *Child*.
Equally, you can substitute a pose in the first sequence for one in
the same position in the second sequence—the *Palm Tree* instead of
the *Triangle*, for example—and vice versa. Check the pages that
describe the individual poses for any tips for beginners. For
instance, you may not feel able to manage the full *Cobra* or
Pose of Tranquillity, but will still benefit from doing the first
two steps. Always start and end in a posture of relaxation,
such as the *Corpse*, for five minutes.

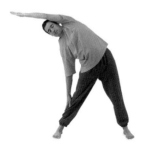

THE PALM TREE
page 104

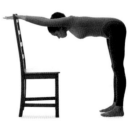

SIMPLE FORWARD BEND
page 106

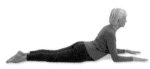

THE COBRA
pages 78–79

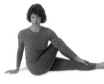

SIMPLE SPINAL TWIST
pages 94–95

THE HERO
pages 88–89

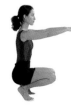

SQUATTING BALANCES
pages 142–143

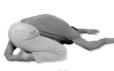

THE HARE
page 63

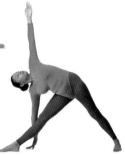

THE TRIANGLE
pages 70–71

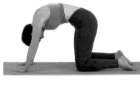

THE CAT
pages 72–73

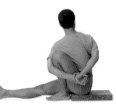

THE SIMPLE SAGE
pages 96–97

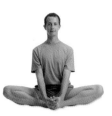

THE COBBLER
pages 84–85

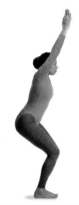

THE POWERFUL POSE
page 109

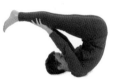

THE POSE OF TRANQUILLITY
pages 148–149

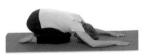

THE CHILD
page 62

Program 2

This is a slightly more advanced program than the first one.
If some of the poses seem too difficult, but you're confident about
others, you can substitute poses from the same position in the list
for the first program—the *Hare* instead of the *Quarter Headstand*
and the *Simple Sage* instead of the *Reverse Sage*, for example. Check
the pages that show the postures in the previous chapter for hints
and tips, such as using your hands to support your back in the
Bridge or learning the full *Squatting Balances* with the aid of a
folded rug. The first seven poses—the *Dog*, the *Back Stretch*, the
Bridge, the *Supine Twist*, the *Eagle Arms Pose*, the *Tree*, and the
Quarter Headstand—form one sequence that can be practiced
independently or that can precede the second sequence—the
Gate, the *Standing Forward Bend*, the *Half Locust*, the *Reverse Sage*,
the *Half Shoulder Stand*, the *Squatting Balances* and the *Head of a
Cow*. The second sequence can also be practiced independently.
Always start and end in a posture of relaxation, such as
the *Corpse*, for five minutes.

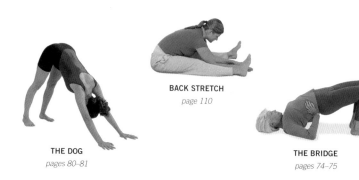

THE DOG
pages 80–81

BACK STRETCH
page 110

THE BRIDGE
pages 74–75

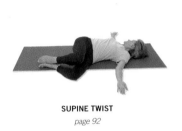

SUPINE TWIST
page 92

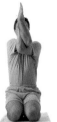

THE EAGLE ARMS POSE
page 120

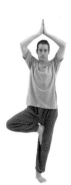

THE TREE
pages 66–67

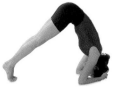

QUARTER HEADSTAND
pages 154–155

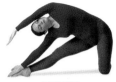

THE GATE
pages 90–91

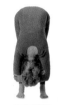

**STANDING
FORWARD BEND**
page 107

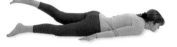

THE HALF LOCUST
page 77

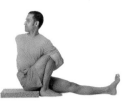

THE REVERSE SAGE
pages 98–99

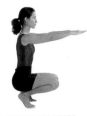

SQUATTING BALANCES
pages 142-143

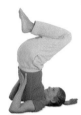

HALF SHOULDER STAND
page 150

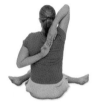

THE HEAD OF A COW
page 83

Program 3

This program incorporates some of the poses already included in the first two programs. There are also some intermediate poses, but if you don't feel ready to try these, you can substitute from the previous programs in the same way as before. The first sequence is the *Warrior,* the *Head–Knee Position* (substitute an easier forward bend if you like), the *Crescent Moon* (or an easier backward bend), the *Revolving Abdomen,* the *Hero,* the *Triangle,* and the *Hare.* The second sequence is the *Tree,* the *Half Boat* (substitute an easier forward bend if you like), the *Basic Fish,* the *Cross-Legged Twist,* the *Classic Thunderbolt,* the *Cobbler,* and the *Wide Legs Posture* (or an easier inverted pose). Always start and end in a posture of relaxation, such as the *Corpse,* for five minutes.

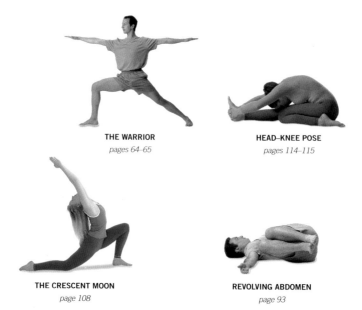

THE WARRIOR
pages 64–65

HEAD–KNEE POSE
pages 114–115

THE CRESCENT MOON
page 108

REVOLVING ABDOMEN
page 93

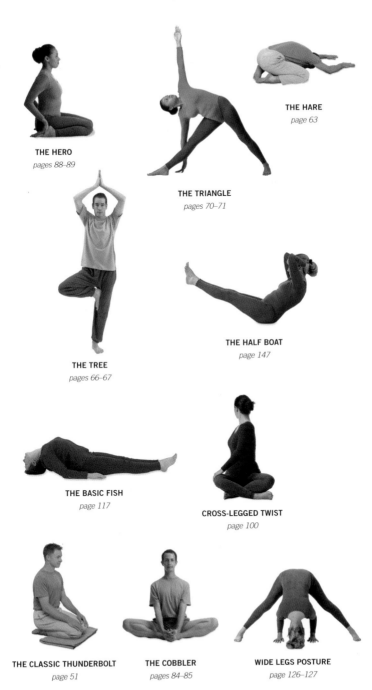

THE HERO
pages 88–89

THE TRIANGLE
pages 70–71

THE HARE
page 63

THE TREE
pages 66–67

THE HALF BOAT
page 147

THE BASIC FISH
page 117

CROSS-LEGGED TWIST
page 100

THE CLASSIC THUNDERBOLT
page 51

THE COBBLER
pages 84–85

WIDE LEGS POSTURE
page 126–127

Program 4

More intermediate poses are included in this program, although there are still some that are suitable for beginners. As before, you can substitute from the previous programs if some of these seem too difficult or you haven't yet learned them. Equally, if there are poses that you feel very confident about, check the pages on which they are described in the previous chapter to see if there is a variation or a further step to offer a little more challenge.

For example, once you can manage the *Simple Spinal Twist* smoothly and easily, you might like to try the *Half Spinal Twist*. The first sequence consists of the *Eagle*, the *Back Stretch*, the *Boat with Oars*, the *Simple Spinal Twist*, the *Classic Thunderbolt*, the *Powerful Pose*, and the *Shoulder Stand*. The second sequence comprises the *Half Moon*, the *Standing Forward Bend*, the *Side Dog*, the *Supine Twist*, the *Easy Position*, the *Squatting Balance*, and the *Quarter Headstand*. Always start and end in a posture of relaxation, such as the *Corpse*, for five minutes.

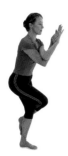

THE EAGLE
pages 68–69

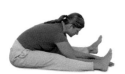

BACK STRETCH
page 110

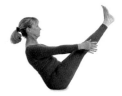

THE BOAT WITH OARS
page 147

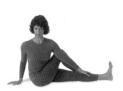

SIMPLE SPINAL TWIST
pages 94–95

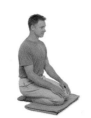

THE CLASSIC THUNDERBOLT
page 51

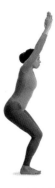

THE POWERFUL POSE
page 109

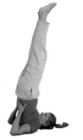

SHOULDER STAND
page 150

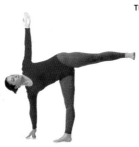

THE HALF MOON
pages 134–135

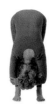

**STANDING
FORWARD BEND**
page 107

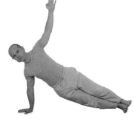

THE SIDE DOG
page 141

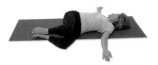

SUPINE TWIST
page 92

EASY POSITION
page 50

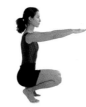

SQUATTING BALANCES
pages 142–143

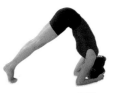

QUARTER HEADSTAND
page 154

Program 5

This is quite a demanding program that will be suitable if you have been practicing regularly and have achieved a good level of flexibility, strength, and stamina. However, the poses from the earlier programs (some of which are included here) and the programs themselves are still valuable and beneficial. Apart from anything else, they are ideal for routine practice when you are concentrating on learning a new pose. As before, you can substitute from earlier programs. The first sequence consists of the *Stretched Side Angle*, the *Half Boat*, the *Cross-Legged Fish*, the *Reverse Sage*, the *Hero*, the *Half Lotus Standing*, and the *Plow*; and the second sequence of the *Wide Legs Posture*, the *Triangle*, the *Bridge*, the *Lunge Twist*, the *Easy Position*, the *Heron*, and the *Crane*. Always start and end in a posture of relaxation, such as the *Corpse*, for five minutes.

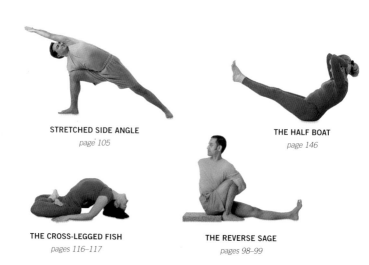

STRETCHED SIDE ANGLE
page 105

THE HALF BOAT
page 146

THE CROSS-LEGGED FISH
pages 116–117

THE REVERSE SAGE
pages 98–99

THE HERO
pages 88–89

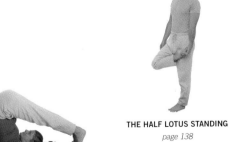

THE HALF LOTUS STANDING
page 138

THE PLOW
page 151

WIDE LEGS POSTURE
pages 126–127

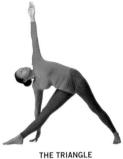

THE TRIANGLE
pages 70–71

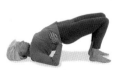

THE BRIDGE
pages 74–75

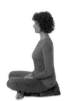

EASY POSITION
page 50

LUNGE TWIST
pages 128–129

THE HERON
pages 118–119

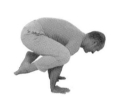

THE CRANE
pages 144–145

Program 6

Although none of the poses in this final program is, strictly speaking, advanced, they all require quite a high level of strength, flexibility, stamina, and, above all, concentration. (You should, of course, concentrate whatever the pose and however easy it is, or you will not be able to do it properly.) It must be emphasized again that you should not force yourself into a pose that you do not feel ready for—this program is not a goal to be achieved. As before, you can substitute poses from the earlier programs. The first sequence is the *Gate,* the *Triangle Forward Bend,* the *Camel,* the *Mermaid,* the *Hero,* the *Heron,* and the *Shoulder Stand* or, perhaps, one of its variations. The second sequence is the *Warrior Lunge,* the *Angled Back Stretch,* the *Wheel,* the *Head of a Cow,* the *Half Lotus,* the *Powerful Pose,* and the *Elbow Stand.* Always start and end in a posture of relaxation, such as the *Corpse,* for five minutes.

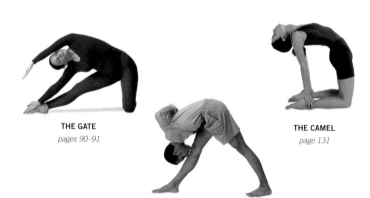

THE GATE
pages 90–91

TRIANGLE FORWARD BEND
pages 102–103

THE CAMEL
page 131

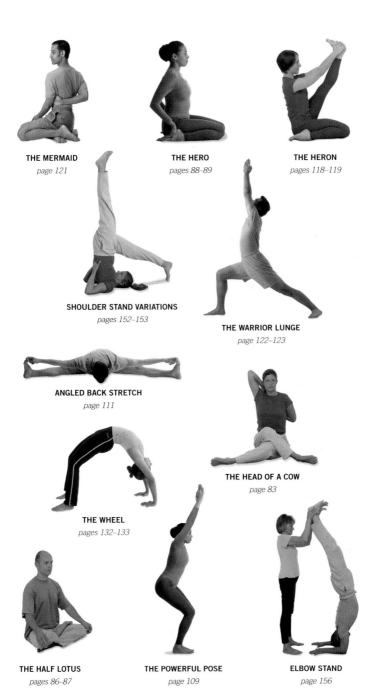

THE MERMAID
page 121

THE HERO
pages 88–89

THE HERON
pages 118–119

SHOULDER STAND VARIATIONS
pages 152–153

THE WARRIOR LUNGE
page 122–123

ANGLED BACK STRETCH
page 111

THE HEAD OF A COW
page 83

THE WHEEL
pages 132–133

THE HALF LOTUS
pages 86–87

THE POWERFUL POSE
page 109

ELBOW STAND
page 156

Hints and Tips

- Try to schedule a regular time, two or three hours after eating, for your yoga practice.
- Pay attention to your body and never force yourself to try poses that are uncomfortable or cause pain. If any of them do, stop immediately.
- Always start and finish each session with a period of relaxation.
- Always do at least five minutes, preferably ten, of warm-up exercises before you start.
- Twists or stretches to one side should always be countered with the same movement to the other side. Forward bends should always be countered with backward bends.
- Finish the session before fatigue sets in. You should feel refreshed both mentally and physically at the end of the session.
- Don't set schedules or targets for "achieving" particular positions.
- Use a folded rug as extra cushioning for inverted poses and, if necessary, for kneeling postures. There is no merit in suffering.

ASTANGA YOGA

Also known as power yoga, *Astanga* yoga has enjoyed a meteoric rise in popularity in the West in recent years, not least because of its endorsement by high-profile pop and movie stars. It is a very dynamic form of exercise, linking postures with jumps and using powerful breathing techniques. It tends to appeal particularly to competitive high-achievers, and some gyms and centers market their classes in a somewhat unscrupulous fashion, suggesting instant fixes. As it uses a set sequence of moves and postures, it is attractive to those who want to practice yoga at home. When done properly, it offers the same kinds of benefits as Hatha yoga, improving physical and mental well-being and fitness. If you want to learn Astanga yoga, it is essential to attend a class taught by a properly qualified teacher, rather than to attempt it on your own, because the risk of injury is considerable.

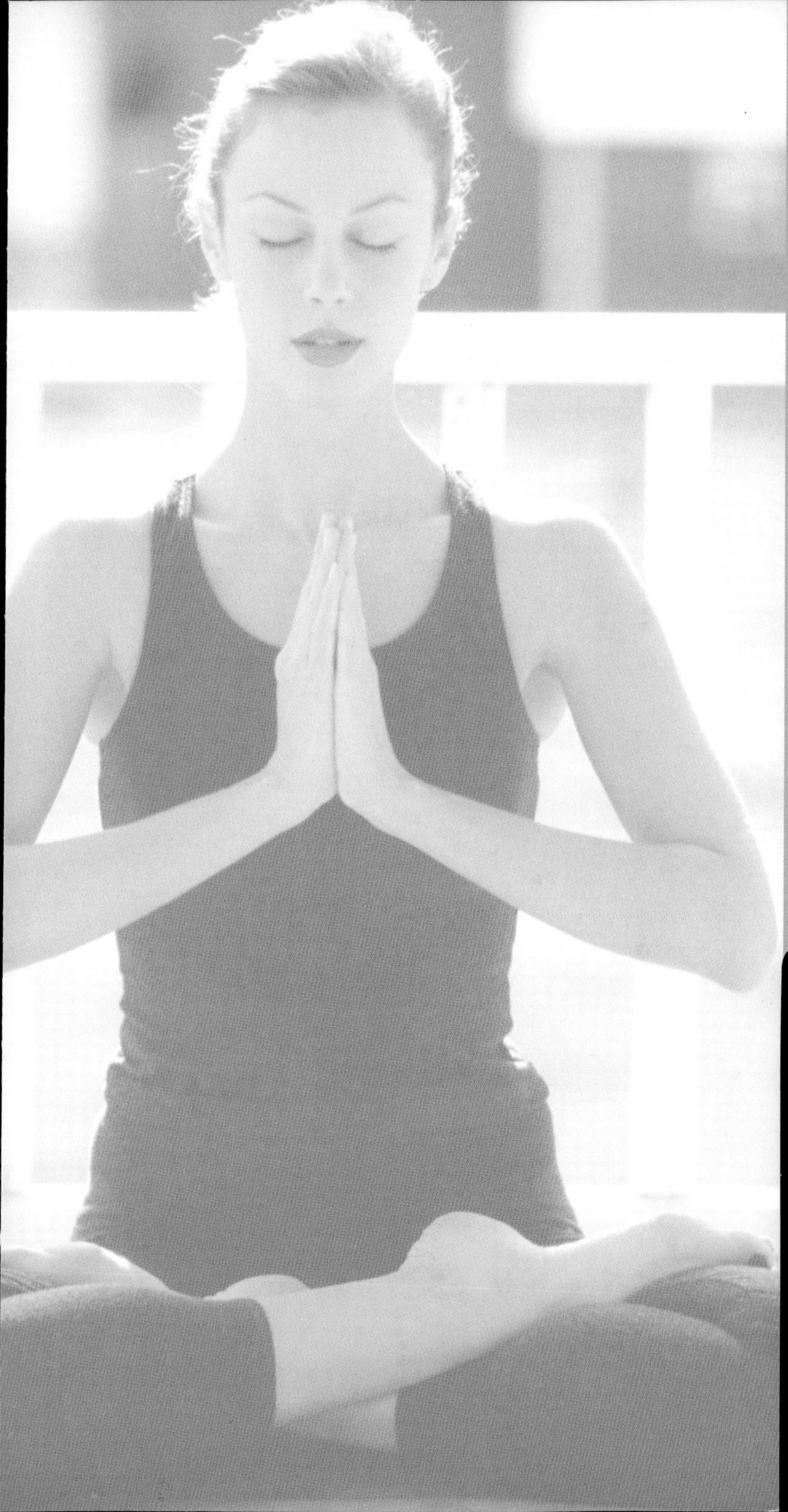

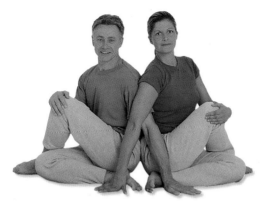

Yoga and Your Lifestyle

One of the great thing about yoga is that you can benefit from it, whoever you are—young or old; fit or out of condition; working or unemployed; thinker or doer; man, woman, or child. You can also use its techniques to make your daily life easier, more pleasurable, and even safer. Stressed in the office? A few simple stretches and some controlled breathing will restore your equilibrium. Worried about a long drive? Ease the tension in your back and shoulders and keep alert with some roadside yoga. First-time granny? By the time he's a toddler, you can have practiced enough yoga to keep up with your energetic grandchild and to look too young to have one.

Everyday Yoga

Self-discipline is required in all aspects of our lives—it's part of what makes us get out of bed to go to work or keep our patience when our two-year-old throws a temper tantrum in a supermarket—but it doesn't come easily to most of us. Practicing yoga is an ideal way of enhancing this quality and creating the serenity of mind to cope with the wear and tear of daily life. Even on a very basic, practical level, sitting down and planning your yoga program for the week is an exercise in self-discipline. It will also help you maintain your initial enthusiasm and resist the temptation to give up because you don't have time, it's too difficult, or you have to finish redecorating the kitchen, wait until the children have started school, lose weight—or any other excuse.

Scheduling your yoga program into your diary may encourage you to keep up regular practice and prevent mundane concerns from nudging it into the background of your life.

One of the best ways of ensuring that you don't lose heart or momentum when you take up yoga is to join a class. This not only guarantees that you are taught the poses correctly, but provides the support of working with other students, who may also become new friends—an extra benefit. There is a huge number of classes available in the daytime, including lunchtime, and evening, and some even provide a crèche. An increasing number of companies offer a lunchtime or after-work yoga class to their employees and there are also physiotherapists who work with yoga teachers to aid recovery after an injury or assist with chronic problems and other special needs. However, before joining a class, do check that the teacher has an accredited qualification.

Never having enough time is the theme song of the twenty-first century, so apply a little lateral thinking. For example, practicing yoga with your partner has extra benefits, reinforcing the bond between you and, quite probably, enhancing your sex life. A busy mum can have quality time with the children in a family yoga session. There are some mother-and-toddler yoga classes, which children usually really enjoy and which counteract the passive and sedentary habit of television. If you are going to practice yoga with a child, you should consult a teacher first, as young bones are still developing and an injury may not become apparent immediately.

Of course, to benefit fully from yoga requires regular practice. It is not necessary to devote hours of every day to it, unless, of course, you want to, but it is worth considering starting each morning with the *Salute to the Sun* (*see pages 58–59*), even if your regular practice is only once or twice a week. Not only will this stretch the spine and limbs and stimulate the circulation, but it will invigorate and energize you for the day ahead and create a positive frame of mind. Think of it as a concentrated yoga program.

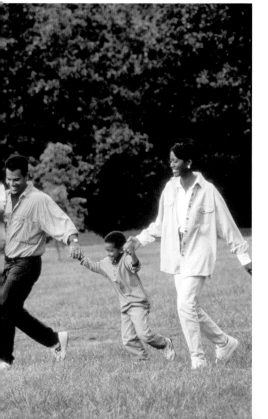

The benefits of yoga will extend into all parts of your life because your improved physical and emotional well-being will enhance your relationships with family, friends, and colleagues.

Yoga for Vitality

Because a balanced yoga program will stretch the spine, tone the muscles and joints of the body, increase the circulation, and encourage proper breathing, virtually all yoga practice promotes vitality. Nevertheless, some postures are particularly energizing and revitalizing. Backward bends, such as the *Half Locust* (see page 77) and the *Cobra* (see pages 78–79), not only stretch the spine, but also stimulate the circulation, providing the spinal nerves with a rich supply of blood. In addition, they open up the chest to improve breathing. Inverted postures, such as the *Hare* (see page 63), stimulate the flow of blood to

The *Warrior* is a dynamic pose that helps develop a positive frame of mind and a sense of control.

the spine, face, scalp, and brain, making you feel and look good. Side stretches, such as the *Warrior* (see pages 64–65), also revitalize the nerves and stimulate the circulation to all the body's organs and tissues. The *Salute to the Sun* (see pages 58–59), especially if you pay attention to your breathing, is a wonderful sequence of movements for getting the energy flowing. Complete the sequence several times on both sides for maximum effect. Don't overlook the value of breathing exercises (see pages 42–45), which clear the mind and also energize the body.

The *Cobra* is an especially good pose for non-pregnant women to practice, as it is very beneficial to the reproductive organs.

Simple Standing Stretch

A healthy spine is the key to feeling fit and well. This simple stretch loosens tension and increases the blood flow to the nervous system, leaving you feeling refreshed and invigorated.

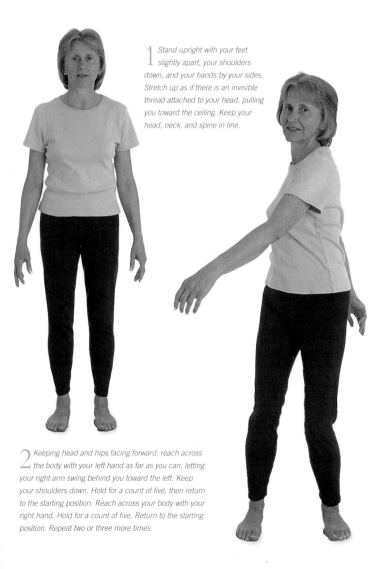

1 *Stand upright with your feet slightly apart, your shoulders down, and your hands by your sides. Stretch up as if there is an invisible thread attached to your head, pulling you toward the ceiling. Keep your head, neck, and spine in line.*

2 *Keeping head and hips facing forward, reach across the body with your left hand as far as you can, letting your right arm swing behind you toward the left. Keep your shoulders down. Hold for a count of five, then return to the starting position. Reach across your body with your right hand. Hold for a count of five. Return to the starting position. Repeat two or three more times.*

Flat Twist

This basic twist stimulates the circulation and helps eliminate toxins, leaving you feeling refreshed and invigorated. Stretching out like a starfish expands the heart and induces feelings of happiness. You may not be able to achieve the full stretch to begin with, but your flexibility will increase with practice.

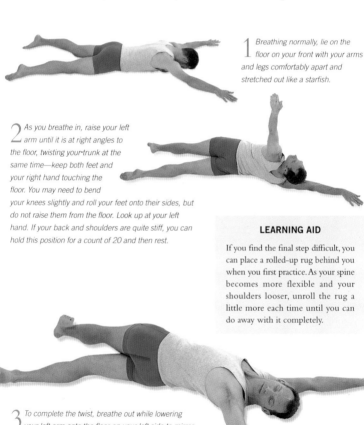

1 Breathing normally, lie on the floor on your front with your arms and legs comfortably apart and stretched out like a starfish.

2 As you breathe in, raise your left arm until it is at right angles to the floor, twisting your trunk at the same time—keep both feet and your right hand touching the floor. You may need to bend your knees slightly and roll your feet onto their sides, but do not raise them from the floor. Look up at your left hand. If your back and shoulders are quite stiff, you can hold this position for a count of 20 and then rest.

LEARNING AID

If you find the final step difficult, you can place a rolled-up rug behind you when you first practice. As your spine becomes more flexible and your shoulders looser, unroll the rug a little more each time until you can do away with it completely.

3 To complete the twist, breathe out while lowering your left arm onto the floor on your left side to mirror the starfish pattern of your arms in Step 1. Do not move your feet or right arm. Try to lower your shoulder to the floor, then stretch and hold the position for at least a count of 30. Return to your starting position, then repeat, raising your right arm and twisting to the right.

Supine Knee Squeeze

Here, the knees are gently squeezed against the body, stretching the muscles of the lower back, limbering the legs, and massaging the abdominal organs. Whether the pose deserves its alternative name of *Wind-Relieving Posture* is debatable, but it certainly benefits the digestive system and is said to help relieve constipation. Although this is quite a gentle stretch, it invigorates the nervous system and leaves you feeling refreshed and energized.

1 *Lie flat on your back on the floor with your knees bent and your feet flat on the floor hips-width apart. Place your hands, palms downward, flat on the floor by your sides. Stretch your spine without arching your back and press your back into the floor.*

2 *Raise your left knee toward your head and clasp your leg just below your knee with both your hands. Do not raise your head from the floor. Pull your left leg toward you as high and as close to your body as you comfortably can. Breathing normally, hug your knee and hold the position for a count of ten, then relax the pressure, but do not move for a count of ten. Squeeze your knee again and hold for a count of ten. Return to your starting position and repeat, raising and squeezing your right leg.*

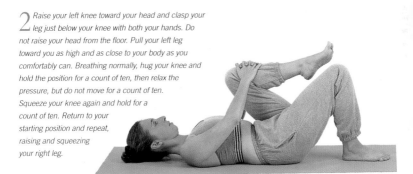

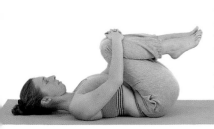

3 *Finally, raise both knees and grasp them with both hands, keeping your back flat on the floor and without raising your head. Breathing normally, hug your knees and hold the position for a count of ten, then relax the pressure, but do not move for a count of ten. Squeeze your knees again and hold for a count of ten. Return to your staring position and repeat, if you like.*

Yoga in the Workplace

It is rarely practical to attempt a full session of yoga in your workplace, as there is unlikely to be sufficient space and your colleagues will probably think you are eccentric, if not certifiably mad. You could take your yoga mat to a quiet place in a nearby park during the summer, but even then you are likely to gather an audience of curious observers. However, you can use yoga techniques to counteract the physical and mental stresses of the working day. Several of the warming-up exercises, such as the head and neck rolls, shoulder shrugging, shoulder rolls, stretching the arms, and flexing the fingers and the feet (*see pages 54, 55, 56, and 57*), are ideal for easing stiffness and tension in a mainly sedentary job. The hand and finger exercises are especially useful for anyone who spends long hours at a keyboard. The *Simple Forward Bend* (*see page 106*) can be managed fairly discreetly without alarming your colleagues and will relieve an aching back resulting from sitting or standing for long periods. Both this bend and the *Palm Tree* (*see page 104*) help to boost the circulation and re-energize a sluggish body and mind. Many of the suggestions for Yoga on the Move (*see pages 184–187*) are also suitable for the workplace. Regular breaks from the computer screen to rest the eyes are recommended by health and safety authorities, and it is good idea to use these as an opportunity to stretch the spine.

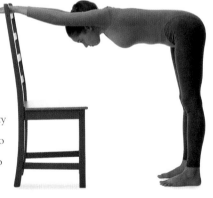

Are You Sitting Comfortably?

Practicing yoga regularly will already have improved your posture and there is no doubt that sitting in the correct way can preempt many tiresome aches and pains. It is essential that your chair is adjusted to the correct height and provides support for your back. Raise the seat of the chair so that your hips are slightly higher than your knees when you sit with your feet flat on the floor. Sit back in the chair with your head, neck, and spine in line. The best office chairs have an adjustable lumbar support that is designed to fit into the curve of your lower back, but if you don't have one, you may find a small cushion helpful. Whatever kind of chair it is, don't perch on the edge of it, as you will inevitably begin to slouch forward. Place your feet flat on the floor hips-width apart. If you are working at a computer, the top of the screen should be level with your eyes when you are looking straight ahead. The monitor and keyboard should be positioned directly in front of you to avoid constant turning and twisting of the neck and shoulders.

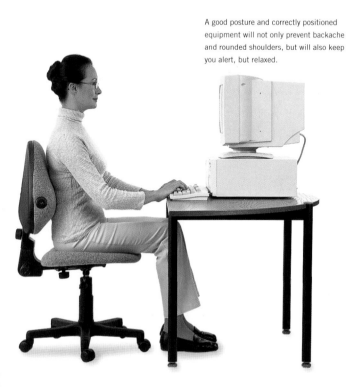

A good posture and correctly positioned equipment will not only prevent backache and rounded shoulders, but will also keep you alert, but relaxed.

Office Yoga Postures

You can easily adapt a number of basic yoga postures to stretch your
back, ease tension in your shoulders, and loosen your spine. Push
your chair back from your desk if you are going to remain seated.

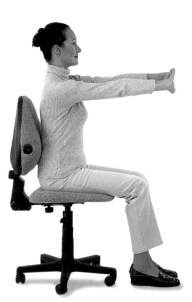

Upstretched Arms

This is a variation of a standing pose and, if you
prefer, you can stand in the *Upright Steadiness*
(*see page 51*). Interlace your fingers and rest
them, palms downward, in your lap. Raise your
trunk from your hips, keeping your head, neck,
and spine in line. Raise your arms, with your
fingers still interlaced, until they are level with
your shoulders. While breathing in, push your
palms away from you. Hold your breath and hold
the position for a count of five, then breathe out
and lower your palms to your lap. Repeat four
more times. Then repeat again, but raising your
arms over your head, and remembering to keep
your shoulders down and level.

Easy Forward Bend

This is a very gentle back stretch, which
provides many of the same benefits as the
head–knee floor poses but to a lesser extent.
Sit toward the front of your chair with your
feet flat on the floor and your hands resting
on your knees. While breathing in, raise
your trunk from your hips with your head,
neck, and spine in line. Tuck your chin into
your chest and, while breathing out, slowly
curl forward, keeping your abdominal muscles
tense. Let your arms stretch down between
your knees. Breathing normally, hold the
position for a count of ten. Then, while
breathing in, gradually unroll until you are
seated upright again. Do not sit up in a hurry.

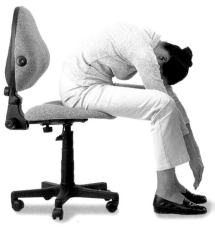

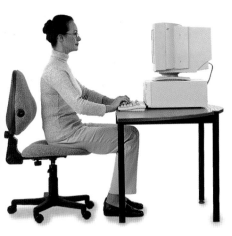

Seated Backward Bend

This is an unobtrusive way to stretch the spine and stimulate the circulation. Sit on your chair with your feet flat on the floor and your head, neck, and spine in line. Raise your trunk from your hips, then tilt your hips forward so that your back is arched. Tense your abdominal muscles and tilt your hips back to the starting position. Keep your shoulders relaxed and don't hunch them as you tilt your hips back. Repeat five times.

The Small Palm Tree

As its name implies, this is a variation of the *Palm Tree* posture (*see page 104*), and you can also do it standing. Sit on your chair with your feet flat on the floor and your head, neck, and spine in line. While breathing in, raise your trunk from your hips, then link your hands and raise them above your head. While breathing out, bend to the right without twisting your hips or shoulders. Breathing normally, hold the position for a count of ten. Then, while breathing in, return to an upright seated position. Repeat nine more times, alternating the direction.

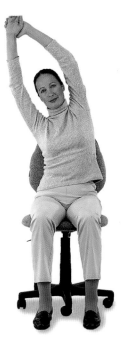

Seated Spinal Twist

An office version of the *Simple Spinal Twist* (*see pages 94–95*), this helps to loosen tension in the back and make the spine more elastic. It also helps to calm the nervous system. Sit on your chair with your feet flat on the floor and your head, neck, and spine in line. Without twisting your hips, grasp the left side of the chair back with your right hand and rest your left hand on the back of the chair. Keeping your shoulders as level as possible, twist your body further to the left by pulling against the chair back with your right hand. Hold the position for a count of ten, then turn to face forward. Repeat, twisting to the right.

Yoga on the Move

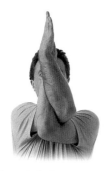

You can do the *Eagle Arms Pose* even in confined spaces to ease tension in shoulders and arms.

Besides transporting you from A to B, cars, trains, and planes all have one thing in common—you sit for a prolonged period in a restricted space. Muscles and joints stiffen, drivers' shoulders become tense, long-haul flights carry the risk of deep-vein thrombosis (DVT), and delays or traffic jams sour your mood. If this isn't bad enough, you are probably also breathing polluted or recycled air. It is no wonder that incidents of road and air rage are becoming more frequent.

When traveling by car, you can stop and get out—take a break every two hours in order to stay alert, and to stretch your limbs. Try to find a quiet place away from the main road. To relieve backache and muscle tension, try the warming-up stretches (*see pages 52–53*), the *Palm Tree* (*see page 104*), and the *Standing Forward Bend* (*see page 107*). *Alternate Nostril Breathing* (*see page 44*) will help restore your equilibrium. Note that passengers practicing postures other than flexing the feet and hands are a driving hazard.

Train, coach, and air passengers may benefit from some of the warming-up exercises, including the head and neck rolls, shoulder shrugging, shoulder rolls, stretching the arms, and flexing the fingers and feet (*see pages 54, 55, 56, and 57*). On long journeys, it is vital to flex the feet frequently to boost the circulation and avoid DVT. The *Eagle Arms Pose* (*see page 120*) is good for loosening the shoulders. Remember too that many of the suggestions for Yoga in the Workplace (*see pages 180–183*) can be adapted for traveling. For example, if space is very limited, clasp your elbows rather than interlace your fingers for the *Upstretched Arms*.

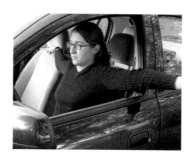

Regular stops on long car journeys keep you alert and enable you to stretch stiff muscles.

Calming Breath

Fear of flying is very common and even frequent fliers sometimes have butterflies in the tummy during take-off and landing. Combining rhythmical breathing with a mantra can calm your mind.

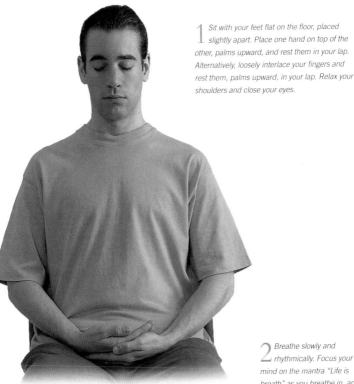

1 *Sit with your feet flat on the floor, placed slightly apart. Place one hand on top of the other, palms upward, and rest them in your lap. Alternatively, loosely interlace your fingers and rest them, palms upward, in your lap. Relax your shoulders and close your eyes.*

2 *Breathe slowly and rhythmically. Focus your mind on the mantra "Life is breath" as you breathe in, and "breath is life" as you breathe out. Focus your concentration on the mantra and the regular rhythm of your breathing.*

COUNTING

You can continue rhythmical breathing and focussing on the mantra until the plane is safely in the air. Indeed, use this technique at any time when you feel the need to calm your mind. It doesn't matter how many times you mentally repeat the mantra, but some people find that counting on a string of *mala* beads is an extra help. There are 108 beads on the string, rather like a rosary. Hold the beads in your right hand and count them between your thumb and middle finger.

Rock and Roll

Traveling puts strain on the lower back, especially when
movement is very restricted. This tilt helps to stretch and loosen
the aching muscles. Passengers can do it at any time and drivers
will find it very helpful during rest breaks.

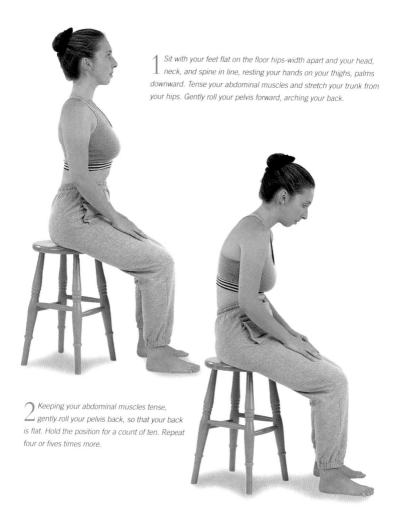

1 Sit with your feet flat on the floor hips-width apart and your head,
neck, and spine in line, resting your hands on your thighs, palms
downward. Tense your abdominal muscles and stretch your trunk from
your hips. Gently roll your pelvis forward, arching your back.

2 Keeping your abdominal muscles tense,
gently roll your pelvis back, so that your back
is flat. Hold the position for a count of ten. Repeat
four or fives times more.

The Traveler's Twist

Car drivers, in particular, will find this helpful for relieving
tension in the neck and spine. Airplane passengers also tend
to become stiff, as movement is very restricted and they are often
quite cramped. It is a good way of improving the flexibility of
the spine and shoulders in general.

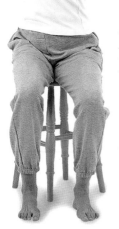

1 Sit toward the front of your
seat with your feet flat on
the floor hips-width apart and
your head, neck, and spine in
line. Place your hands on your
shoulders with your elbows out
to the sides. Stretch your trunk
up from your hips. Then, while
breathing in, push your left
shoulder forward and your right
shoulder back without twisting
your hips or neck.

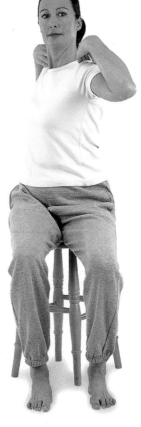

2 Twist as far to the right as you comfortably
can, leading with your left shoulder and
keeping both shoulders down. Breathing normally,
hold the position for a count of ten, then slowly
return to your starting position. Repeat, pushing
your right shoulder forward and your left shoulder
back. Then repeat on both sides twice more.

Yoga with Your Partner

It has been reported that people's sex lives have gained vitality and their pleasure has been enhanced when one partner practices yoga, and this effect is even more marked when both do. This is partly a result of improved muscle tone, more supple joints, increased vitality, and an overall feeling of well-being. It is also due to the fact that practicing yoga eases tension and anxiety, increases concentration, and opens the mind to being more responsive.

Therefore, it is not necessary to understand or practice Tantric yoga to benefit in this way, because it is a serendipitous side effect of practicing Hatha yoga. However, some postures are thought to be particularly valuable for improving sexual vigor, increasing the health of the reproductive system and sex glands, and developing a flexible spine and supple hips. These include the *Classic Thunderbolt* (*see page 51*), the *Cobra* (*see pages 78–79*), the *Locust* (*see page 77*), the *Bow* (*see page 130*), the *Shoulder Stand* (*see page 150*), the *Plow* (*see page 151*), and the *Simple Spinal Twist* (*see pages 94–95*). In addition, *bandhas*— techniques for temporarily blocking the passage of air through the lungs—are thought to harness sexual energy and do act directly on the sexual organs.

It has been emphasized throughout this book that yoga is non-competitive. Nor, of course, should lovemaking be competitive, but people do worry about their "performance" or whether they compare favorably to a previous partner. Practicing yoga together is the perfect way to dispel these damaging anxieties and to enhance your physical and emotional intimacy.

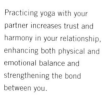

Practicing yoga with your partner increases trust and harmony in your relationship, enhancing both physical and emotional balance and strengthening the bond between you.

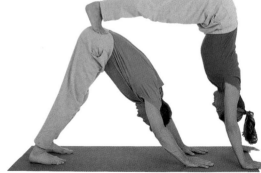

Double Spinal Twist

This pose increases spinal flexibility and relieves tension, including headaches. It also massages the abdominal muscles and dispels sluggishness. You start back to back and, as you become more supple, the further you can twist and the closer the two of you become. Beginners can practice a simple version, while those with more flexible spines can try the slightly more advanced pose.

1 Sit on the floor back to back with your legs in front of you and spines in line. Raise your trunk up from your hips. Bend the knee of your outer leg (here, he bends his left knee and she bends her right). Clasping your knee with your hands, place your foot flat on the floor beside the outside of the thigh of your inner leg.

2 Still clasping your raised knee, place the outer hand (his left, her right) flat on the floor beside your partner's bottom—do not lean on it. Breathing out, turn the shoulders, as far as you comfortably can, toward your outer hand—do not lift your bottom off the floor, and keep the back straight. Breathing normally, hold for a count of ten. Relax and repeat on the other side.

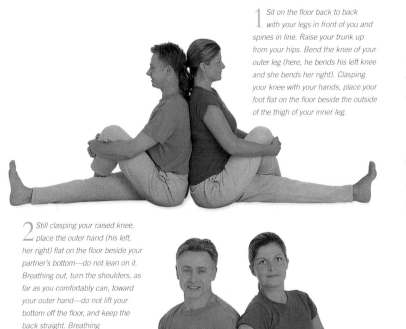

The Simple Warrior in Pairs

This full body stretch raises your energy levels and increases vitality. Working with your partner helps to enhance strength, stamina, coordination, and balance, as well as increasing closeness. Take turns to steady each other.

1 *Stand in the* Upright Steadiness *(see page 51) facing each other an arm-length apart. Breathing normally, raise your arms above your head, keeping your shoulders down, then place your hands, palms downward, on your partner's shoulders. Keeping your head, neck, and spine in line, transfer your weight to your right foot. While breathing in deeply, extend your left leg behind you until it is straight, "locking" your right knee. Breathe out.*

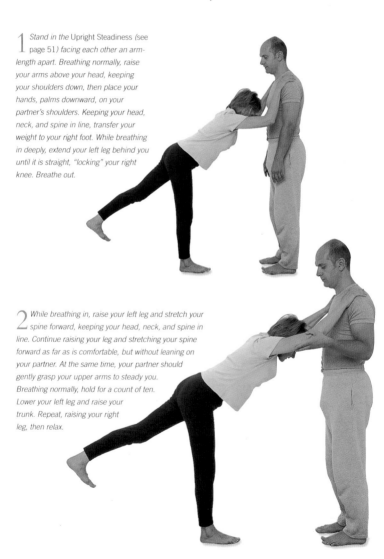

2 *While breathing in, raise your left leg and stretch your spine forward, keeping your head, neck, and spine in line. Continue raising your leg and stretching your spine forward as far as is comfortable, but without leaning on your partner. At the same time, your partner should gently grasp your upper arms to steady you. Breathing normally, hold for a count of ten. Lower your left leg and raise your trunk. Repeat, raising your right leg, then relax.*

Partner Squat

This posture is a true test of a balanced relationship and, to begin with, is harder than it looks, as one partner is likely to be stronger than the other. It improves balance and concentration and strengthens the feet, knees, and thighs.

1 *Stand in the* Upright Steadiness *(see page 51) facing each other. Raise your arms in front of you and clasp your partner's hands. Move your feet hips-width apart. While breathing in deeply, rise up on your toes.*

2 *While breathing out and still balancing on your toes, squat down, keeping your head, neck, and spine in line. Do not let your knees swing apart and keep both arms straight. Lower your heels and hold the position for a count of at least six. While breathing in, stand up, still holding your partner's hands and keeping your arms straight.*

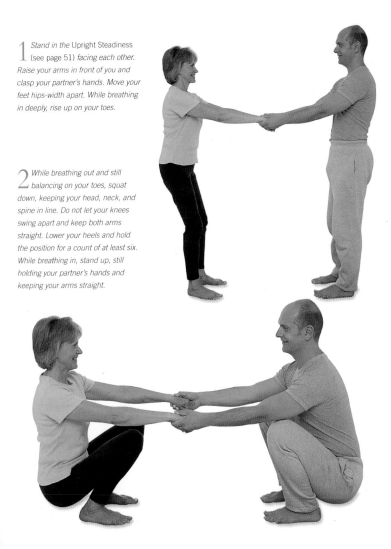

Yoga to Keep You Young

People who have practiced yoga throughout most of their lives and continue to do so in their sixties, seventies, and beyond may have suppleness, stamina, lissomeness, and good health that are the envy of others half their age. As well as increasing the flexibility of the spine, toning muscles, and limbering the limbs, yoga raises energy levels, balances hormones, boosts the immune system, and encourages healthy circulation of blood and oxygen to all the tissues of the body. In addition, practicing yoga maintains or restores confidence, which is so easily and frequently undermined by the negative attitude toward aging in the West.

Use a foam block to help keep your spine straight and increase the stretch when first practicing sitting twists.

Taking up yoga in middle age or later is very beneficial, as long as you approach it in a sensible way. When you have done little or no exercise for maybe 30 years, your joints will have stiffened, your spine will have lost its flexibility, and your muscles will lack tone. You may also have acquired a lifetime's bad habits and poor posture. Start with simple poses and take your time to practice and perfect them. Don't feel that you are "giving in" if you use a cushion, folded rug, or foam block to help when you are learning poses, such as the *Classic Thunderbolt (see page 51)* and *Cross-Legged Twist (see page 100)*, or use a belt for practicing the *Tree (see pages 66–67)*. Keep your movements smooth and flowing, because jerking into a pose is harmful to joints and muscles at any age. Be aware of your body's capabilities and progress at your own pace. Equally, don't dismiss yourself as too old to try if you feel that you can learn a particular pose. Yoga may not put years on your life, but it can put life in your years.

You can use cushions or a folded rug to ease the stress on creaking knees if you are not used to kneeling.

Standing Forward Bend

This helps to mobilize the joints and make the spine more elastic. It also increases the blood supply to the brain and invigorates the nervous system. This is a variation on a pose that is a more gentle stretch of the hamstrings and spine. Stop if you experience pain.

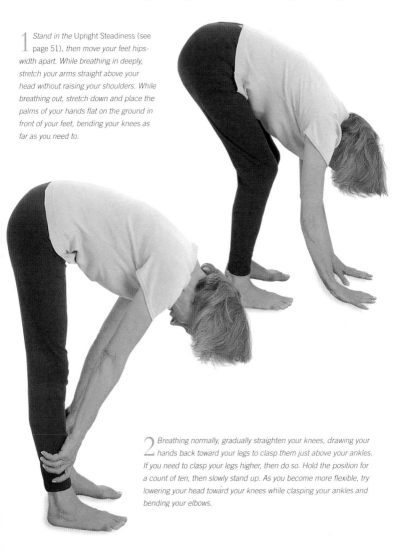

1 *Stand in the* Upright Steadiness (see page 51), *then move your feet hips-width apart. While breathing in deeply, stretch your arms straight above your head without raising your shoulders. While breathing out, stretch down and place the palms of your hands flat on the ground in front of your feet, bending your knees as far as you need to.*

2 *Breathing normally, gradually straighten your knees, drawing your hands back toward your legs to clasp them just above your ankles. If you need to clasp your legs higher, then do so. Hold the position for a count of ten, then slowly stand up. As you become more flexible, try lowering your head toward your knees while clasping your ankles and bending your elbows.*

Alternating Stretch

This strengthens the muscles of the abdomen and back and
promotes balance and coordination. It tones the legs and
shoulders, leaving you feeling invigorated and rejuvenated.

1 *Start on all fours with your knees hips-width apart. Angle your
hands slightly inward and straighten your arms without "locking"
your elbows. Focus your gaze on place between your hands and tuck
in your chin slightly. Breathing normally, extend your left leg behind
you and raise it as high as is comfortable without twisting your hips.*

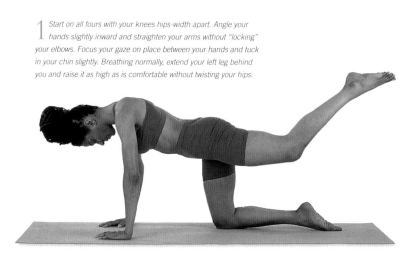

2 *Keeping your chin tucked in, raise your right arm until level with
your shoulder. Stretch your arm away from your shoulder and your
leg away from your hips. Hold the position for a count of five, then
lower your arm and leg. Repeat, stretching your right leg and left arm.*

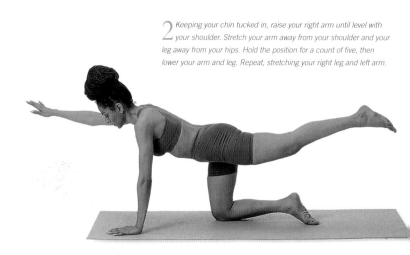

Gentle Triangle Forward Bend

This is a wonderful boost to the circulation, increasing energy levels and dispelling sluggishness. It increases the flexibility of spine and shoulders and relieves tension.

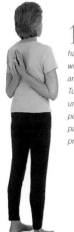

1 *Stand upright with your feet hips-width apart. Place your hands together behind your back with your fingertips touching and pointing downward. Turn your hands inward until your fingers are pointing upward and the palms of your hands are pressed together.*

2 *With hands in the Prayer position (see page 58) or elbows clasped behind you, take a small step forward with your right leg and balance your weight evenly. Lift your trunk up from your hips and comfortably stretch forward, keeping your knees straight. Hold the position for a count of five, then return to your starting position and repeat stepping forward on your left leg.*

Gentle Back Bend

This is an energizing pose, increasing the blood flow to the spinal column, helping to rejuvenate the nervous system.

2 *While breathing in, raise your head and move your arms so that your elbows are directly beneath your shoulders, your forearms flat on the floor. In a continuous movement, raise your shoulders and chest from the floor. Hold the position for a count of ten, then return to your starting position.*

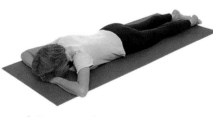

1 *Lie prone on the floor, turning your head sideways and resting it on your hands. Your legs should be straight out behind you, but relaxed, with the toes pointing inward and the heels out to the sides.*

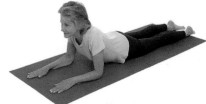

Overcoming Stress and Fatigue

Stress can be very damaging—initially you may not even be aware that you are stressed. If you are subjected to prolonged stress, you may start to recognize what is happening, not least because of feelings of fatigue. It is tempting to adapt to living in this state rather than tackling the causes. This cannot go on forever without resulting in ill health and complete exhaustion.

The best way to deal with stress is to nip it in the bud, and regular yoga practice is a good way of doing this, as it calms the mind, refreshes the body, and restores a sense of balance and harmony. Use the relaxation positions (*pages 60–63*) and the *Pose of Tranquillity* (*pages 148–149*) to unwind after a busy day or before sleep. Ironically, the more you suffer from fatigue, the more likely you are to develop insomnia. You may find meditation or visualization techniques helpful in overcoming this.

Tension accumulates in the shoulders, neck, and back, so poses that stretch, tone, and loosen these areas are very useful. These include backward bends, such as the *Bridge* (*see pages 74–75*) and the *Cobra* (*see pages 78–79*); forward bends, such

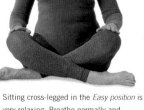

as the *Back Stretch* (*see page 110*) and the *Simple Forward Bend* (*see page 106*); and spinal twists, such as the *Simple Spinal Twist* (*see pages 94–95*) and the *Supine Twist* (*see page 92*). Inverted poses, such as the *Dog* (*see pages 80–81*), are very calming. Breathing techniques (*see pages 42–45*) help restore balance.

Don't let your yoga practice become another stress. If this is happening, the worst thing you can do is give up. Instead, concentrate on poses that you can manage comfortably and smoothly. Leave learning new postures until you are feeling less stressed.

Sitting cross-legged in the *Easy position* is very relaxing. Breathe normally and concentrate on the pattern of your breathing.

Relaxation

Take time to unwind by relaxing in one or all of the following poses. Close your eyes and focus on your breathing.

Corpse with Knees Bent

This is a good position for practicing visualization before going to sleep at night. Lie flat on your back with your hands at your sides, palms upward. Stretch out your legs, then bend your knees, drawing your feet toward you. Bring your knees together and turn your toes slightly inward. Breathe deeply for several minutes.

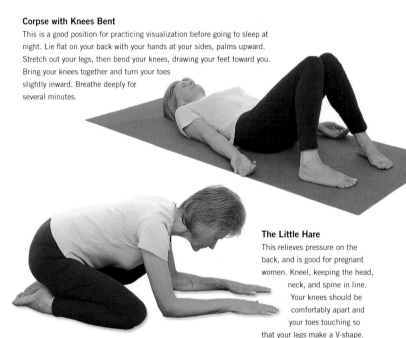

The Little Hare

This relieves pressure on the back, and is good for pregnant women. Kneel, keeping the head, neck, and spine in line. Your knees should be comfortably apart and your toes touching so that your legs make a V-shape. Lowering your bottom onto your heels, place your elbows on the floor beneath your shoulders. Breathe deeply for several minutes.

Rescue Position

This is the perfect position for sleeping, as it is relaxing, and doesn't encourage snoring. Lie down on your right or left side (whichever is more comfortable), and rest your head on a pillow so that your head, neck, and spine are in a line. If you are lying on your right side with your right cheek on the pillow, bend your right leg slightly and bring your left knee over to rest on the floor. Bend your elbows and rest your left hand and forearm on top of your right.

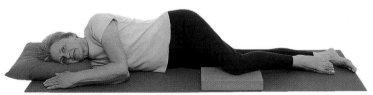

Leg Stretch

This is a very relaxing and restorative posture that acts as a pick-me-up when you are feeling stressed and tired. It is an easy pose to learn without adding to your stress, and using the wall as a support makes it even more relaxing. When you feel comfortable with this pose, you can do it without the extra support.

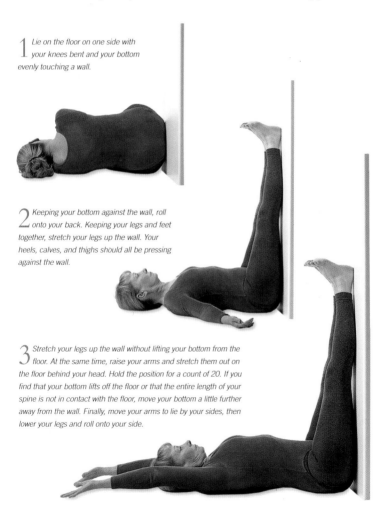

1 Lie on the floor on one side with your knees bent and your bottom evenly touching a wall.

2 Keeping your bottom against the wall, roll onto your back. Keeping your legs and feet together, stretch your legs up the wall. Your heels, calves, and thighs should all be pressing against the wall.

3 Stretch your legs up the wall without lifting your bottom from the floor. At the same time, raise your arms and stretch them out on the floor behind your head. Hold the position for a count of 20. If you find that your bottom lifts off the floor or that the entire length of your spine is not in contact with the floor, move your bottom a little further away from the wall. Finally, move your arms to lie by your sides, then lower your legs and roll onto your side.

The Rolling Plow

Inverted poses, where your head is lower than your heart, are excellent for overcoming fatigue, as they stimulate the circulation, particularly to the brain. Tucking in the chin in this pose stimulates the thyroid gland, which produces a hormone to combat fatigue. It also loosens the spine and relieves tension in the shoulders.

1 Lie flat on your back with your head, neck, and spine in line. Bend your knees and place your feet together flat on the floor. Bring both your knees toward your chest and clasp your hands behind them, keeping your bottom on the floor.

2 Gradually straighten your legs until your feet are above your head, sliding your hands along your lower legs to your ankles. You will need to raise your bottom to do this, but your shoulders and back should remain flat on the floor.

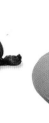

3 Still clasping your ankles, gradually lower your feet to the floor behind your head, lifting your hips and lower back to do so. Keep your legs together and as straight as possible. This should be a smooth movement—don't tug your ankles.

THE CHIN LOCK

This bandha, or lock, is very beneficial if you are suffering from fatigue. Sit or stand with your head, neck, and spine in line. Breathe in and hold your breath. Press your chin down into your chest between your collar bones. Hold the position, then raise your chin while breathing out. Stop if you feel dizzy and do not practice this if you have an overactive thyroid.

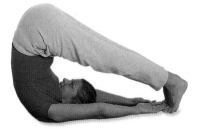

4 Tuck your toes under to point at your head and stretch your arms, palms upward, to touch your toes. Hold as long as you can. Roll back, reversing each step. Relax in the Corpse (see page 60).

Yoga and Common Ailments

Although yoga is not a therapy, it can assist both the healing and prevention of many common ailments. It is not a substitute for conventional treatment and you should check with your physician first.

- **Asthma** the Bow (*see page 130*), the Cobra (*see pages 78–79*), the Corpse (*see page 60*), the Basic Fish (*see page 117*), the Hare (*see page 63*), the Half Locust (*see page 77*), the Locust (*see page 77*), the Palm Tree (*see page 104*), the Shoulder Stand (*see page 150*), the Supine Twist (*see page 92*)

- **Backache** the Back Stretch (*see page 110*), the Bow (*see page 130*), the Bridge (*see pages 74–75*), the Cat (*see pages 72–73*), the Cobra (*see pages 78–79*), the Basic Fish (*see page 117*), the Head of a Cow (*see page 83*), the Simple Spinal Twist (*see pages 94–95*)

- **Bronchitis** the Bow (*see page 130*), the Basic Fish (*see page 117*), the Half Locust (*see page 77*), the Locust (*see page 77*), the Palm Tree (*see page 104*)

- **Cellulite** the Eagle (*see pages 68–69*)

- **Constipation** the Back Stretch (*see page 110*), the Cat (*see pages 72–73*), the Basic Fish (*see page 117*), the Head–Knee Pose (*see pages 114–115*), the Plow (*see page 151*), the Simple Forward Bend (*see page 106*), the Simple Spinal Twist (*see pages 94–95*), the Stretched Side Angle (*see page 105*), the Supine Knee Squeeze (*see page 179*), the Triangle (*see pages 70–71*)

- **Fatigue** *see pages 196–199*

- **Flatulence** the Squatting Balances (*see pages 142–143*), the Supine Knee Squeeze (*see page 179*)

- **Indigestion** the Bow (*see page 130*), the Cobra (*see pages 78–79*), the Corpse (*see page 60*), the Half Locust (*see page 77*), the Locust (*see page 77*), the Plow (*see page 151*), the Pose of Tranquillity (*see pages 148–149*), the Simple Spinal Twist (*see pages 94–95*), all simple standing stretches

- **Insomnia** the Back Stretch (*see page 110*), the Cobra (*see pages 78–79*), the Corpse (*see page 60*), the Half Locust (*see page 77*), the Locust (*see page 77*), the Plow (*see page 151*), the Pose of Tranquillity (*see pages 148–149*)

- **Liver problems** the Boat with Oars (*see page 147*), the Half Boat (*see page 147*), the Revolving Abdomen (*see page 93*), the Simple Spinal Twist (*see pages 94–95*)

- **Menstrual problems** the Cat (*see pages 72–73*), the Cobra (*see pages 78–79*)

- **Overweight** the Back Stretch (*see page 110*), the Bow (*see page 130*), the Cobra (*see pages 78–79*), the Head-Knee pose (*see pages 114–115*), the Revolving Abdomen (*see page 93*), the Simple Forward Bend (*see page 106*), the Simple Spinal Twist (*see pages 94–95*), the Standing Forward Bend (*see page 107*), the Stretched Side Angle (*see page 105*), the Triangle (*see pages 70–71*)

- **Piles** the Dog (*see page 80–81*), the Basic Fish (*see page 117*), the Plow (*see page 151*), the Shoulder Stand (*see page 150*)

- **Rounded shoulders** the Basic Fish (*see page 117*), the Camel (*see page 131*)

- **Rheumatism** the Back Stretch (*see page 110*), the Cobra (*see pages 78–79*), the Head of a Cow (*see page 83*), the Head-Knee pose (*see pages 114–115*), the Simple Spinal Twist (*see pages 94–95*), the Triangle (*see pages 70–71*)

- **Sciatica** the Back Stretch (*see page 110*), the Half Locust (*see page 77*), the Locust (*see page 77*)

- **Stress** *see pages 196–197*

- **Thyroid problems** the Bridge (*see pages 74–75*), the Basic Fish (*see page 117*), the Shoulder Stand (*see page 150*)

- **Varicose veins** the Half Locust (*see page 77*), the Locust (*see page 77*), all inverted postures

Glossary

Words in italics have individual glossary entries.

Asana Sanskrit word meaning pose or posture.

Astanga yoga Based on Raja yoga, this is a very dynamic form of power yoga.

Atman The Self.

Bandha Muscular lock.

Bhakti yoga Devotional yoga, involving practices such as prayer and chanting.

Brahman The Absolute, Oneness, the Divine.

Chakras Energy centers to which the *nadis* channel *prana*.

Chin Mudra The hand position in which the thumb and index finger are joined.

Hatha yoga A mainly physical form of yoga, using *asanas* and *pranayama*. It also incorporates other principles, such as meditation and spiritual enlightenment.

Ida One of the three most important *nadis*.

Jnana yoga The yoga of philosophy and self-knowledge.

Karma Sanskrit word meaning action applied to the principle of cosmic cause and effect.

Karma yoga The yoga of spiritual action and the selfless service to humanity.

Mala A string of 108 beads used for counting, rather like a rosary.

Mandala Circular symbol of unity and wholeness.

Mantra A word or phrase repeated mentally or out loud to focus the mind.

Nadis Channels through which *prana* travels to the *chakras*.

Namaste The Prayer position, in which the palms of the hands are placed together with the fingers pointing upward.

Niyamas Observances.

Om The universal mantra, representing the Absolute. Sometimes Aum.

Pingala One of the three most important *nadis*.

Prana Cosmic energy or the life force.

Pranayama Breathing exercises designed to cleanse and strengthen the mind and body by controlling the flow of *prana*.

Rajas The quality of overactivity, energy, and passion.

Raja yoga Scientific yoga.

Sattva The quality of purity, intelligence, order, and light.

Sushumna One of the three most important *nadis*.

Sutra A thread, used to describe an explanatory technique of a series of highly condensed statements.

Tamas The quality of inertia, resistance, laziness, and lethargy.

Yamas Abstinences.

Useful Addresses

UNITED STATES

Sivananda Yoga Vedanta Center
243 West 24th Street
New York
New York 10011
Tel: 212 255 4560
www.sivananda.org

Sivananda Yoga Vedanta Center
1200 Arguella Boulevard
San Francisco
California 94122
Tel: 415 681 2731
www.sivananda.org

The Yoga Alliance
234 South 3rd Avenue
West Reading
Pennsylvania 19611
Tel: tollfree 1-877-YOGAALL
  964 2255 or 610 376 4421
www.yogaalliance.org

The Yoga for Health Foundation
7918 Bolling Drive
Alexandria
Virginia 22308

CANADA

The Yoga for Health Foundation
1562 Southdown Road
Mississanga
Ontario L5J 2Z4

The Yoga for Health Foundation
2121 Galena Crescent
Oakville
Ontario L6H 4A9

UNITED KINGDOM

British Wheel of Yoga
1 Hamilton Place
Boston Road
Stanford
Lincolnshire NG34 7ES
Tel: 01529 306851
www.members.aol.com/wheelyoga

Sivananda Yoga Vedanta Centre
51 Felsham Road
London SW15 1AZ
Tel: 020 8780 0160
www.sivananda.org

The Yoga for Health Foundation
Ickwell Bury
Biggleswade
Bedfordshire SG18 9EF
Tel: 01767 627271
www.yogaforhealthfoundation.co.uk

For general information contact
www.yogasite.com

Further Reading

Laurent de Brunhoff
Babar's Yoga for Elephants
Abrams, 2002

David Fontana
A Meditator's Handbook, A
   Comprehensive Guide to Eastern
   and Western Meditation Techniques
Element Books, 1998

Richard Hittleman
Yoga: A 28-Day Exercise Plan
Bantam, 1998

Stella Weller
Yoga Therapy: Safe Natural Methods
   to Promote Healing and Restore
   Health and Well-Being
Thorsons, 1998

B. K. S. Iyengar
Tree of Yoga
Aquarian Press, 1998

Stephen Sturgess
The Yoga Book
Element Books, 1997

Howard Kent
Breathe Better Feel Better
Apple Press, 1997

B. K. S. Iyengar
Light on Yoga
Schocken, 1996

Swami Vishnudevananda
The Complete Illustrated
   Book of Yoga
Yes International, 1996

Silvia Klein Olkin
Positive Pregancy Fitness
Avery Publications, 1996

**Miriam Friedman and
   Janice Hankee**
Yoga at Work
Element, 1996

Howard Kent
The Complete Yoga Course
Headline, 1993

Swami Prabhavananda
Spiritual Heritage of India
Vedanta Publications, 1993

Howard Kent
Yoga for the Disabled
Sunrise Publications, 1985

Index

Many thanks to all the yoga

models who feature in this book

and special thanks to Joanne Avison

for her sound advice.